Management of Minor Head Injuries

Management of Minor Head Injuries

I.J. Swann
MB, BS, FRCS (Eng)
Consultant in Accident and Emergency Medicine
Glasgow Royal Infirmary
Hon. Clinical Lecturer
Glasgow University

and

D.W. Yates
MA (Cantab.), MCh (Orth.), FRCS
Senior Lecturer in Accident and Emergency Medicine
University of Manchester
Hon. Consultant
Accident and Emergency Department
Hope Hospital, Salford

MEDICAL LIBRARY
W   GENERAL HOSPITAL

LONDON
Chapman and Hall Medical

First published in 1989 by
Chapman and Hall Ltd
11 New Fetter Lane, London EC4P 4EE

© 1989 Chapman and Hall Ltd.

Typeset in 11/13pt Palatino by
Best-set Typesetter Limited, Hong Kong

Printed in Hong Kong

ISBN 0 412 29080 4

British Library Cataloguing in Publication Data

Swann, I. J.
    Management of minor head injuries.
    1. Man. Head. Injuries. Therapy
    I. Title II. Yates, David W. (David William)
    617'.51044

    ISBN 0-412-29080-4

Contents

Preface

In the United Kingdom about one out of every ten new patients attending an Accident and Emergency (A and E) Department has a head injury. Some are severely injured on presentation, others deteriorate hours or even days later. In the vast majority the incident is not very serious and these patients are allowed home on the same day or after a short period of observation. However, the diagnosis of 'mild head injury' can only be made in retrospect and initial treatment must reflect concern about the development of complications. This book is about the early management of all these patients and for the definitive care of the largest group in which mild head injury may be the cause of prolonged morbidity.

It is aimed at junior medical staff but the contents will also be of value to nurses who work in the A and E Department or Observation Ward. It is intended to be of particular use to doctors who wish to gain information rapidly 'on the shop floor'. The first two chapters deal with clinical assessment and documentation of findings. Advice on resuscitation is included as the apparently mild head injury may in itself be potentially lethal or may present in combination with other life-threatening injuries.

The third chapter discusses the merits of investigations including C.T. scanning and skull radiography. The criteria for radiography and admission have been developed from experience in A and E Departments in busy city hospitals with ready access to X-ray facilities and observation beds but are recommended for use in any district general hospital.

The practical aspects of scalp wound management and local anaesthetic technique are covered in Chapter 4. Nowadays, particular care in wound exploration and suturing is necessary not only for the patient's benefit but also for the surgeon's own protection. Every doctor and nurse should consider completing a course of Hepatitis B immunisation before starting work in the A and E Department.

Occasionally patients who are thought to have minor injuries on first examination subsequently require urgent neurosurgical care. Chapter 5 emphasises the need for early identification of these patients by means of well-defined routines for observation and referral. The exceptional case for emergency intra-cranial surgery in a referring hospital is discussed. For this very rare occasion facing the inexperienced surgeon, the technique for making burr-holes is described.

Throughout the text reference is made to the peculiarities of presentation, the difficulty of assessment and the special needs of young children. Particular attention is also paid to the elderly, the epileptic, the drug abuser, and the intoxicated patient.

Doctors working in A and E Departments frequently comment that they do not get enough feedback about the recovery of patients that they have treated. It is not generally appreciated that a mild head injury can cause protracted social and medical problems for patient and family. These late neurological and psychological sequelae are discussed in Chapter 6, which describes how the outcome depends not only upon the early management but also most importantly upon subsequent rehabilitation measures.

Ian Swann, Glasgow

David Yates, Manchester

Foreword

A million people come every year to Accident and Emergency (A and E) departments in Britain after recent head injury, almost half of them children. Most are only mildly injured but among these are a few who develop complications. By producing secondary brain damage these can threaten life or lead to life-long disability. That is why these patients, who account for about 10% of new attenders at A and E departments, cause such concern to the doctors who have to decide about their management. In many American emergency departments this problem is often resolved by a neurosurgical consultation – because the hospitals have neurosurgeons on their staff. In almost all other countries the responsibility for the initial care of all head injuries, and for the whole care of the mildly injured falls on other specialists – A and E doctors, general or orthopaedic surgeons, or paediatricians. The care of head injured patients would improve if more of these doctors were better informed about head injuries, and had clearer ideas about their management. Ensuring that the many head injuries that are initially mild are competently managed would be likely to save more lives, and to prevent more disability, than focusing most attention on patients who have already sustained severe brain damage.

The development of A and E medicine as a specialty, with many consultants appointed and more in approved training programmes, has transformed the organization and standard of care in many A and E departments. Several of these consultants have recognized that mild head injuries present an interesting challenge – not only initially but until they have recovered. However, the majority of patient contacts are inevitably with relatively junior doctors – either those training to be A and E specialists, or those who are rotating through A and E departments as part of training for other branches of medicine. Because head injuries are so numerous these doctors and their nursing colleagues need a pragmatic text that makes it clear what they ought to do. This book does that and it provides a basis for constructing local guidelines, in collaboration with the staff of the regional neurosurgical unit. These should declare explicitly what each specialist expects of the other, in the best interests of all head injured patients.

A short practical book cannot be expected to deal with the prevention of head injuries, but the importance of this should not be overlooked. Road accidents are a much less frequent cause of the predominantly mild injuries that come to A and E departments than are falls and assaults. Alcohol more often contributes to falls and assaults than it does to mild head injuries resulting from road accidents. Preventive measures should be targeted in these directions, as well as on road safety.

It is to be hoped that this book will make more doctors regard head injuries as interesting and challenging, rather than as a nuisance and a threat. Doctors in A and E departments have much to contribute, not only in triage but in ensuring that the mildly injured, whether admitted briefly for observation or sent home, are adequately followed up. There is much temporary morbidity in the mildly injured that could be reduced if head injured patients were to be more often dealt with by doctors who were well informed and confident about appropriate action and advice.

Bryan Jennett MD FRCS
Professor of Neurosurgery
Institute of Neurological Science
Glasgow
January 1989

Acknowledgements

We thank our colleagues in Glasgow and Manchester who have helped in the preparation of this book. These include all the A and E staff who share their experience of head injury management every day and fellow specialists who have made constructive comments on the text. The Departments of Medical Illustration in our two hospitals have assisted in the preparation of illustrations and our secretaries have typed the manuscript with characteristic skill and good humour. Our wives and publishers have shown great tolerance and patience throughout the project.

We are delighted that Professor Bryan Jennett has enriched the book with his Foreword. It was largely his pioneering work on head injury management which stimulated us to put pen to paper.

1 Presentation

1.1 HISTORY

The great majority of patients who have sustained mild head injuries and some who have sustained more severe damage will be talking more or less coherently by the time they arrive at the Accident and Emergency department. They may therefore be able to give an account of the incident and the subsequent journey to hospital. This may be plausible but is often unreliable. A conversation with a head injury patient some days after the event may reveal a surprising lack of recall of events in the A and E department – despite an apparently normal conversation having occurred at that time. It is wise, therefore, to detain any witnesses and ambulance personnel who may be able to give more precise details of the incident, so that an accurate history can be obtained once initial assessment has been completed.

The patient tends to recall events and actions but have a poor memory of the duration of inactivity. For example, he may remember the circumstances of the accident and of being thrown to the ground. He may then recall getting up immediately and coming to hospital in an ambulance. He may be less clear about how long he had to wait for the ambulance or indeed not recall lying on the ground for some time after being knocked down.

Post-traumatic amnesia (PTA)

This condition is defined as the length of time from the injury to the return of continuous memory. Islands of apparent normality may punctuate this period of amnesia but should not be taken as indicating its termination. It may be difficult to be certain that PTA has indeed resolved when the patient is first seen in the A and E department. A repeat examination some time after the first assessment is usually necessary, with the patient being asked to recall information given at the first examination. Demonstration of an inadequate short-term memory should be taken as indicative of continuation of PTA (Section 2.1). Post-traumatic amnesia correlates directly with the severity of diffuse brain injury and it is therefore valuable to estimate its duration as carefully as possible.

Retrograde amnesia

This term refers to the period of amnesia immediately prior to the accident. This is usually only a few seconds but may be prolonged and out of proportion to other symptoms and signs. Alcohol intoxication may be so severe as to cause genuine amnesia for several hours before the injury. Migraine, hysteria and various psychiatric conditions may have a similar effect. Sometimes retrograde amnesia appears to be influenced by the patient's anxiety about the accident. For example, the patient may feel guilty about being discovered intoxicated or in a socially compromising situation. Alternatively he or she may have been involved in some criminal activity. An artificial extension of retrograde amnesia in such circumstances is a useful alibi. It will be appreciated, therefore, that retrograde amnesia, unlike PTA, is of little value in determining the extent of brain injury.

Circumstantial evidence

Evidence of this type may help to reconstruct the relative movements of the head and the injuring agent so that the biomechanics of impact can be determined. This can be of great help in the assessment of the probable extent of brain injury. Information from police and ambulance staff about the patient's behaviour at the scene and during transport to hospital is of great value. Clinical notes should summarize statements made by the patient and witnesses and not contain value judgements or information unrelated to assessment or management. If the patient is abusive, his or her remarks should be briefly transcribed in quotation without written comment thereon.

Children

Child subjects are particularly difficult to assess. Their immature behavioural res-

ponses and understandable anxiety may produce a wide spectrum of presenting symptoms. Unfortunately the paucity of crisp, clinical evidence of brain injury and even the absence of a skull fracture does not guarantee immunity from an intracranial haematoma. The parents' opinion about the behaviour of their child is particularly important and should always be sought (Section 2.6).

Child abuse

Abuse should be considered if the history given by the parents is unclear or inconsistent with the physical findings. Other suspicious factors include unreasonable delay in presentation, parents displaying disturbed behaviour in the A and E department and evidence of previous abuse within the family. Some A and E departments run an automatic check on recent attendances of siblings of young patients, and all such departments must have 24-hour access to the local 'at-risk' register.

1.2 PREVIOUS HISTORY AND INTERCURRENT ILLNESS

The previous history may be relevant to the cause of and the responses to the injury and can be useful in determining the likely outcome and best management. Patients with bleeding diatheses or on anticoagulant therapy are more liable to develop intracranial haematoma and should be considered at 'Special Risk' (Sections 4.5 and 5.4). Fragile bones increase the risk of skull fracture and those with migraine may suffer an exacerbation following minor head injury. Patients with diabetes mellitus, and those who have abused alcohol or drugs will require continued management of these problems after recovery from the head injury.

Children with headache and vomiting often have coincidental viral infections. The patient, parents and siblings should be asked about coughs, sore throats, diarrhoea, rashes and contact with contagious diseases.

In the elderly there may be a history of dizzy spells, frequent falls and treatment for hypertension. The head injury may have been sustained in a fall caused by the side-effects of medication (Table 1.1; Section 1.4).

It is useful to know the patient's current drug therapy particularly if this includes anticoagulants, antibiotics, steroids, anticonvulsants, antihypertensives and psychoactive drugs. A history of allergy should be sought, in particular to penicillin. Patients with an atopic tendency who suffer from hay fever and sinusitis may develop a frontal headache associated with rhinorrhoea which may be confused with the complications of a fracture of the frontal fossa.

1.3 MECHANISM OF INJURY

An understanding of the biomechanics of the impact can help in the interpretation of symptoms and the assessment of prognosis. Accidents which subject the head to modest deceleration or acceleration forces over a relatively long period of time, such as might occur in a crashing car, tend to produce diffuse axonal injury. When there is a more sudden change of velocity over a shorter time span, as might occur in a fall off a ladder with the head striking the ground, there is a greater likelihood of intracerebral

lacerations and subdural haematoma. Extradural haematoma develops secondarily to direct impact against the skull, when displaced bone tears underlying meningeal vessels.

In both types of accident the mobile head strikes a relatively fixed object and there is therefore a bending or twisting force applied through the neck. This has implications for initial management (Sections 2.3 and 4.1). In contrast, when the relatively stable head is struck by a mobile object (for example a golf club) there is usually little strain on the neck but considerable local damage to the scalp. This may not be associated with a generalized loss of consciousness. However, local skull and brain damage may be severe (Section 2.7).

Road traffic accidents

Victims of road traffic accidents (RTA) should be assumed to have sustained transmitted damage to the cervical spine until proved otherwise. Often the patient has painful limb injuries which divert attention away from the neck. The late development of neck pain after road traffic accidents is discussed in Section 6.2. It is essential to know if the patient was a pedestrian or a vehicle occupant. The position of the latter and information about use of a seat belt, child harness or neck restraint helps in the the appreciation of the forces imposed on the head. In this respect it is useful to know if the vehicle was struck from the front, side or rear and if it remained upright or rolled over and whether or not the patient was ejected. Passengers wearing correctly fitting seatbelts will usually not penetrate the windscreen although flying glass can embed deeply into scalp wounds. The driver's head may, however, make contact with the steering wheel and sustain direct forehead injury. Improvements in steering wheel design (and the introduction of air bags, as in North America) should reduce this type of injury.

Falls

These may cause, or be a consequence of, head injury. A history of epilepsy, alcohol abuse, transient ischaemic attacks, diabetes or simple fainting should be sought. Although these pre-existing conditions may confuse assessment and lead to a prolongation of retrograde amnesia and post-traumatic amnesia, it is wise to ascribe all symptoms to the head injury itself for the purposes of initial management. Witnesses may be particularly helpful in this type of case.

Assault

Assault is usually associated with intoxication both of the perpetrator and the victim. Neither can be relied upon to give an accurate account of the incident. Relatives or colleagues attending the department with the patient may also be biased in their account of the incident. Scalp wounds in assaulted patients must be assumed to be associated with compound depressed skull fractures until the latter are excluded by exploration (Section 4.4) and radiography.

Scalp wounds caused by blunt impact are commonly associated with a period of amnesia but injuries inflicted by heavy knives, swords or choppers may indent the skull without producing amnesia, abnormal

neurological signs or symptoms. There may, however, be a specific neurological deficit. Unless an accurate history has been obtained, this type of injury can be overlooked or underestimated. Inappropriate management may lead to meningitis or cerebral abscess formation. Evidence from the police about the weapon and the manner in which it had been used may help to avoid this problem.

Sport

Sport is a common cause of head injury but unlike assault there are usually plenty of witnesses who can provide an accurate and reliable history. In some 'sports', for example boxing, a doctor may be in attendance and be able to provide a useful account of the incident. In others, such as horse riding or motor racing, safety helmets will usually have been worn. The helmet should be examined together with the patient. There may be evidence of damage to the former but no scalp injury to the latter. In any event the patient must be told to buy a new safety helmet and not to use the damaged one. However trivial the apparent injury to the helmet, it may have been significantly weakened. In the above mentioned sports and in rugby or football accidents the neck may have been injured at the same time as the head.

The euphoria and machismo associated with sporting activities encourages the player to continue the game after sustaining a minor head injury. Those responsible for the safety and care of their teams should discourage this impulse. Apparently trivial head injuries can impair high-level mental and physical function for several weeks and the effects can be cumulative if multiple minor injuries are sustained.

Scalp wounds sustained in outdoor sporting accidents should be assumed to be contaminated even if on initial inspection they appear to be linear and clean. 'Hit with a golf club' should prompt the diagnosis of compound depressed skull fracture until proven otherwise by wound exploration and skull radiography.

1.4 SYMPTOMS

Headache

This is by far the commonest symptom associated with a recent head injury, occurring in about one-third of adults and one in ten children [1, 2]. There are two types. A well-localized pain may be due to a scalp contusion or laceration. This may be associated with a skull fracture. The second type is less well-defined and not localized on scalp palpation. This type is more likely to be of intracranial origin and if persistent or severe suggests the possibility of raised intracranial pressure. This is particularly likely if the pain is made worse by coughing or straining. However the majority of headaches are mild and are not in themselves helpful in assessing prognosis. They usually settle within a few days unless the patient has a predisposition to headaches or migraine. The patient who presents the day after an alcoholic binge with a headache should be assumed in the first instance to have significant intracranial pathology and not dismissed with the assumption that he has a 'hangover'.

Pain at the back of the head may arise from neck strain. This is discussed in Section 6.2. Severe headache associated with neck stiffness, photophobia and a positive Kernig's sign is more likely to be due to a traumatic subarachnoid haemorrhage than neck strain (Section 2.6). The management of patients who present with persisting headaches is discussed in Section 6.2.

Nausea and vomiting

These symptoms are particularly common in drunks and young children after head injury. One out of every 13 head injured adults vomits before or during assessment in the A and E department, and one in eight complains of nausea. Coincidental illness, inappropriate medication or co-existing abdominal injury increase the probability of vomiting. It is very unusual for vomiting to be the sole indicator of a significant head injury. Persistent vomiting without other signs of head injury can usually be ascribed to pathology elsewhere or to poisoning.

Dizziness and vertigo

Dizziness is a term used by patients to describe a variety of symptoms ranging from minor headache to vertigo. When used correctly, vertigo refers to a subjective feeling of rotation or spinning. If it is brought on or made worse by movement of the head, e.g. looking up or turning suddenly, the vertigo is usually due to a disturbance of the vestibular mechanism. It is often associated with vomiting, unsteadiness and a significant period of post-traumatic amnesia. It may be associated with a fracture of the petrous temporal bone, when tinnitus and hearing loss are also likely to be present. Some patients, particularly the elderly, may have a pre-existing tendency to develop vertigo, unsteadiness or syncope. Table 1.1 summarizes the aetiology of these symptoms.

Visual disturbance

This symptom occurs frequently after deceleration injuries but is usually transient. It is probably caused by an interruption of information processing, the first stage of diffuse axonal injury, in the visual cortex. An expanding intracranial haematoma usually produces additional signs and symptoms, particularly depression of conscious level (Section 2.6).

Diplopia may result from local damage to the extra-ocular apparatus of one eye. There may be generalized bruising or specific trapping of an extra-ocular muscle at a fracture site. Distant cranial nerve damage (for example to the sixth nerve associated with a fracture of petrous temporal bone), will also affect eye movement and cause diplopia. The head injury may upset the precarious muscle balance of a latent strabismus, but this effect is usually temporary.

Blurring of vision in one eye in the fully conscious patient is likely to be due to local damage, e.g. macular oedema. It is important to determine the extent of residual vision by measuring the acuity (Section 2.8). Significant deterioration may indicate an expanding retro-bulbar haemorrhage

Table 1.1 Causes of dizziness in the elderly

Symptom	*Possible causes*
Vertigo (a feeling of rotation or spinning)	Head injury Otitis media Menieres disease Benign positional vertigo Cerebellar haemorrhage Cerebellar tumour Psychogenic
Unsteadiness (of gait)	Chronic subdural haematoma Normal pressure hydrocephalus Acoustic neuroma Diabetes mellitus Alcohol/drugs Cervical spondylosis
Syncope (transient loss of consciousness)	Pneumonia/bronchitis Myocardial infarction Cardiac arrhythmia Carotid sinus syndrome 'Vaso vagal' attack Vertebro-basilar insufficiency

pressing on the optic nerve. This requires immediate decompression by an ophthalmic or other competent surgeon to prevent permanent blindness (Section 2.8).

Fits

These are associated with less than 1% of head injuries but should always be assumed to be a direct result of that head injury until proved otherwise. The history may be vague and of course an epileptic seizure may have preceded the head injury. However, it is usually impossible to obtain an accurate history in such cases and it is best to admit the patient for observation. Details of previous fits and anticonvulsant medication should be sought. Blood levels of drugs such as Phenytoin are valuable in assessing recent compliance with therapy (Section 3.2). The possibility of the fits being related

---

Box 1

CASE HISTORY

A thirty-five year old man was brought by ambulance from the scene of a road traffic accident. The ambulancemen had found him lying unconscious on the floor of the front of a car with his legs on the road. The windscreen had been completely shattered but no other vehicle or object of impact was evident.

His neck was splinted and he was carefully extricated from the vehicle. On the way to hospital he began to talk and localize painful stimuli.

What is the likely mechanism of injury?

A doctor passing the scene within a few minutes of the incident had found the man lying on the floor of the car with both legs sticking upright through the shattered windscreen. He was cyanosed and his neck was twisted, but a good pulse was felt. Holding his jaw forwards restored the airway. His legs were repositioned. He then breathed spontaneously but remained unresponsive for at least ten minutes until the ambulance arrived.

It was subsequently discovered that the man had been drinking heavily and had walked in front of the car, entering it head first. A policeman who was first on the scene was convinced the man was dead. In fact he made a good recovery within twenty-four hours.

Golden rules

1. At a road traffic accident always initiate basic life support even to apparently fatally injured patients.

2. Don't extrapolate mechanisms of injury from fragmented reports by witnesses.

to alcohol, hypoglycaemia or anoxia (sections 4.2 and 4.4) should also be considered. A witness should be asked to describe the type and timing of the seizure and the initial after-effects. This may help to determine immediate and long-term management.

1.5 EXTRACRANIAL INJURY

One-quarter of adults with a post-traumatic amnesia of less than one hour have additional injuries, usually involving the arm and face. These are not always immediately detected as the patient or doctor may be preoccupied with the head injury. However, even if there is primary cerebral injury, the initial assessment must be directed towards preventing secondary brain damage and this includes detecting major injuries. The most important secondary effects are caused by hypoxia and hypovolaemia and therefore attention must be directed towards maintenance of the airway and blood volume (Section 4.1).

The patient's preoccupation with his scalp laceration may distract him from complaining of other apparently less important wounds. Symptoms from these must be sought. This task can be made easier by a better understanding of the biomechanics of the injury which may highlight areas of the body likely to have been damaged. A full physical examination is of course also necessary (Chapter 2).

2 Examination

2.1 INITIAL ASSESSMENT

About 90% of head injured patients will appear to be fully conscious when they first present to the Accident and Emergency department. Much information can therefore be gained before a traditional 'hands on' examination is begun. For example, during the initial introduction the patient should be asked various personal details (e.g. name, address, age) and supplied with any information about the accident that he does not volunteer (e.g. circumstances of accident, name of hospital, time of day). Retention of this information can then be tested some minutes later during the examination. A note should be made of any disparity between the recall of this information (short-term memory) and the recall of personal details (long-term memory). If short-term recall is impaired or the patient is disorientated then it is likely that the eventual assessment of post-traumatic amnesia (PTA) will be longer than that estimated in the Accident and Emergency department. Nevertheless it is useful to record this provisional PTA for comparison with the eventual one which will be obtained some time after admission when continuous memory has been restored.

The patient's gait can be assessed whilst he is moving about the examination room. Normal co-ordination and agility precludes major long tract signs in the lower limbs. Similarly upper limb function can be assessed quickly by asking the patient to hold the arms outstretched with palms facing upwards and eyes tightly closed. This will reveal any facial asymmetry as well as upper limb weakness or loss of proprioception (Fig. 2.1).

The emotional state of the patient will be revealed during this initial assessment. The relative size of the pupils, the presence of scalp lacerations and facial injuries and any restriction of neck movement will also be evident.

2.2 GENERAL EXAMINATION

Extracranial injuries may be obvious or suspected from the nature of the accident. When these are life-threatening, a list of priorities must be drawn up and appropriate treatment begun at once. This is discussed in Chapter 4. In all cases a systemic examination must be carried out to establish baselines and record the presence or absence of damage to each part of the body.

If there is concern about previous health, for example a fall in an elderly patient, then

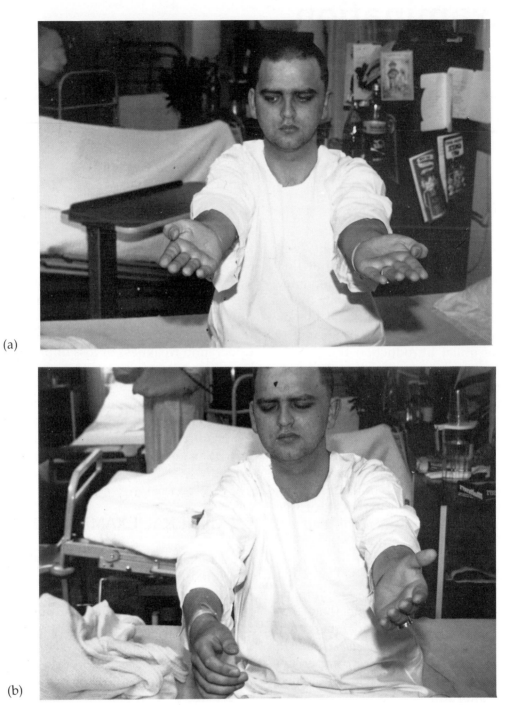

(a)

(b)

Fig. 2.1 Upper limb asymmetry: (a) initial appearance (b) on closing eyes; downward drift and pronation evident after 20 s.

a full examination, particularly of the cardiovascular system, is necessary.

When there is a suspicion of child abuse, a sensitive general examination should be carried out, preferably by a senior member of the A and E department. Admission should be advised on clinical grounds. The possibility of abuse should not be raised with the parents or guardian in the department. This is best left to the paediatrician and social worker once the child has been admitted.

2.3 CERVICAL SPINE

Movement should be formally (but carefully) tested only if the patient is fully conscious and co-operative. Active movements are elicited in flexion, extension, lateral flexion and rotation. No attempt must be made to move the head passively or against pain. The spinous processes should be palpated for irregularity or tenderness and any spasm of the cervical muscles causing abnormal posture noted. If the patient is not fully conscious and co-operative this examination should be deferred and a cervical collar applied.

2.4 THE SCALP

The commonest site for a scalp wound of whatever type is the frontal region. Examination of the scalp from eyebrows to occiput can be carried out conveniently whilst the neck is being examined. Infants should be examined sitting up and if the fontanelles are full in this position then raised intracranial pressure should be suspected.

'Closed' wounds
(bruising, abrasions, etc.)

Soon after injury there may be little to find apart from abrasions, petechiae or tenderness. After a few hours, swelling of the scalp will be more evident. Scalp haematomas become soft as they resolve. Their well-defined raised edge can be mistaken for a depressed skull fracture (Fig. 2.2). In children, if there is associated hair loss, the possibility of abuse should be considered.

Visible bruising and swelling may develop quite quickly around the eyes and ears

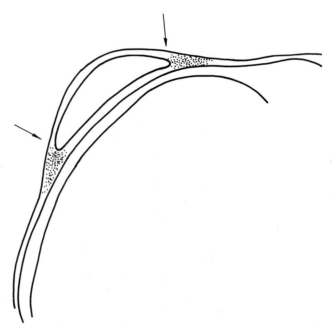

Fig. 2.2 Scalp haematoma simulating depressed vault fracture. Arrows indicate junction of liquified haematoma and consolidated inflammation towards the margin of the 'lump'. Palpation here may give the impression of a vault defect, but the edge is smooth, usually extends around the lesion and is not particularly tender.

following direct trauma. Fracture of the petrous temporal complex on the other hand may lead to the delayed appearance of bruising in the mastoid region (Battle's sign, Section 2.9).

'Open' wounds

It is important to wear gloves for protection when examining any area where there may be bleeding. While searching through the hair look for glass fragments. Once the wound has been identified trim the hair to identify its extent. Note the length of the wound and the nature of the skin edges. Most will be irregular or contused (Fig. 2.3) and only 10–20% will have clearcut incised edges (Fig. 4.4; Section 4.4) [3]. Providing there are no visible foreign bodies in the wound a sterile dressing can be applied prior to X-ray. If there is any doubt about the depth of the wound after initial inspection then definitive exploration should be carried out in sterile conditions. This is discussed in detail in Section 4.4.

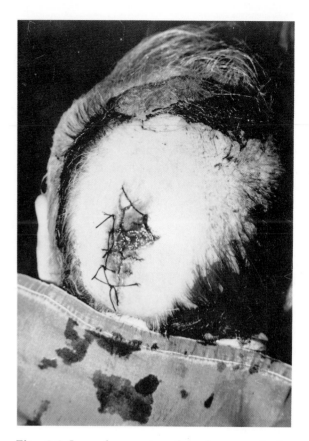

Fig. 2.3 Irregular contused scalp wound. Intoxicated patient fell backwards onto floor.

2.5 THE FACE

Facial fractures may be associated with head injury. However, if the impact is directed only at the face it will absorb considerable energy and this may protect the brain from the major injury which it might have sustained had the blow been directed at the cranial vault.

Nasal bleeding associated with a swollen tender nose is commonly due to direct trauma in which case it will usually stop within a few hours. The isolated nasal fracture is often associated with mild infra-orbital bruising (Fig. 2.4) and occasionally with a septal haematoma which requires urgent drainage.

The more extensive naso-ethmoidal fracture and the much wider complex of injuries (Le Fort types II and III) are usually accompanied by severe peri-orbital bruising, swelling, and after a few hours, by subconjunctival haemorrhage. They may be accompanied by bloodstained CSF rhinorrhoea which, as it runs over the face, may appear as 'tramlines' with blood on either side of the stream of CSF. The Le Fort fractures may be detected by careful palpation of the

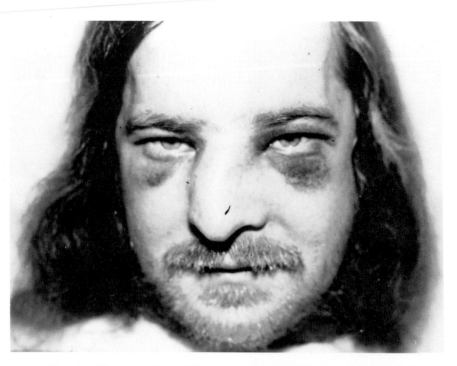

Fig. 2.4 Fractured nasal bones with typical infra-orbital bruising.

facial skeleton and attempted movement of the maxilla against the skull by finger and thumb grasping the incisor area.

A more common injury is a unilateral fracture of the malar complex produced by a direct blow to the cheek, e.g. by fist or boot. This produces local pain and swelling and diffuse bruising spreading to the peri-orbital region. Occasionally an indentation can be seen before the swelling develops (Fig. 2.5).

Most of these fractures of the 'middle third' of the face (maxilla and naso-ethmoidal complex) can be associated with epistaxis, mal-occlusion of the teeth, infra-orbital nerve damage and diplopia (Section 2.8).

Fracture of the body of the mandible is sometimes self-evident but, if not, it should be detected by intra-oral examination (bleeding of gums and sublingual bruising) and testing occlusion, which is painful. Injuries to the condylar neck and temporo-mandibular (TM) joint are more easily missed. The TM joint movement can normally be palpated via the anterior wall of the external auditory canal. Damage to the TM joint can cause bleeding from this anterior wall unlike the petrous temporal fracture of the skull base which usually breaches the posterior or superior wall of the canal.

Traumatic pneumatocoele is an unusual complication of fracture of the frontal, maxillary or ethmoidal air sinuses (Fig. 2.6). The patient presents with unilateral or bilateral peri-orbital swelling of rapid onset which may not be associated with much local bruising or evidence of facial injury. The swelling may enlarge visibly if the patient (unwisely) attempts to blow his

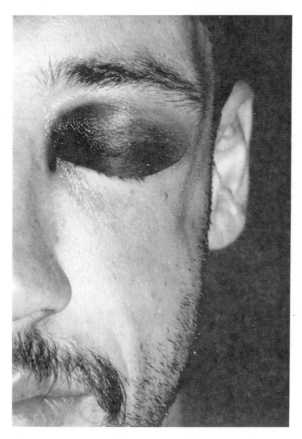

Fig. 2.5 Fracture of malar complex due to karate kick. The indentation is clearly seen.

nose or coughs. Palpation reveals the classical crackling indentation which can be elicited when air is trapped under the skin (surgical emphysema). The same injury may produce an aerocoele (intracranial air). Management is discussed in Section 4.2.

2.6 LEVEL OF CONSCIOUSNESS

Accurate assessment of the level of consciousness is most important both in terms of initial management and prognosis. Normal mentation is the best available clinical indicator of higher cerebral function. Impairment of higher intellectual performance is the earliest sign of deterioration in cerebral function.

Recording the level of consciousness is equally important. Such ambiguous descriptors as stuporose, semi-conscious, obtunded and restless are best avoided. They introduce subjective assessment and significant inter-observer error.

The Glasgow Coma Scale (GCS)

This provides a simple and objective method of expressing the conscious level based on three unambiguous responses – eye opening, motor response and verbal response (EMV). It is described in Table 2.1. It should be noted that discrepancies occur in the published usage of the 'best motor response'. The original publication by Teasdale and Jennett ascribed a score of six to a normal motor response [4]. Some texts have reduced the number of categories in this field to five by combining the 'flexion withdrawal' response with the abnormal flexion of decorticate rigidity. This regrouping is only acceptable if the top motor score remains at six and score four is deleted. Some publications incorrectly renumber the motor scale from one to five thereby reducing the total Glasgow Coma Scale from 15 to 14. This anomaly should be recognized and avoided.

Children

The inability of young children to converse and comprehend limits the usefulness of the GCS in this group. Modifications of the

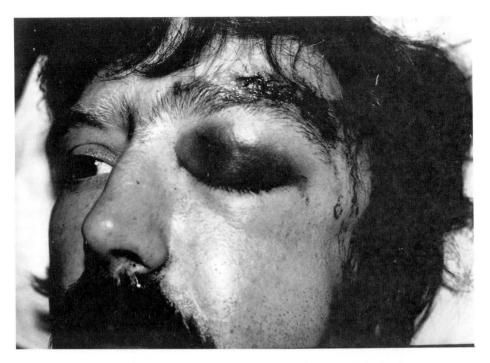

Fig. 2.6 Fracture of left frontal bone with traumatic pneumatocoele.

Table 2.1 The Glasgow Coma Scale

Eye opening (E)	
Spontaneous	4
To voice	3
To pain	2
None	1
Motor response (M)	
Obeys	6
Localizes	5
Withdraws	4
Flexes	3
Extends	2
None	1
Verbal response (V)	
Orientated	5
Confused	4
Inappropriate	3
Incomprehensible	2
None	1

Glasgow Coma Scale are now available and are recommended for use on paediatric observation wards as well as in A and E departments (Section 5.1).

Difficulty is often experienced in scoring a child's eye opening response. Initially the eyes may be closed but will then open as the observer speaks. This gives a theoretical response of E3 – 'eyes open to speech'. It should however be interpreted according to the circumstances. Often it is a normal response for a young child who may usually be asleep at that time of day. If sleep is deep, gentle shaking or a mild stimulus (pinching the earlobe) may be required to obtain eye opening, whereupon the young child may begin talking and playing normally or at least behaving in a way that the parents recognize as normal under the circumstances. This would give a GCS of E2 'eyes open to pain', M6 'plays' and V5 'normal words'.

It is important to use the GCS consistently as described to reflect the conscious level immediately prior to arousal. The decision to discharge a child who was 'sleeping' on arrival at the Accident and Emergency department and one hour later is fully conscious will depend upon other criteria for admission but also upon whether the sleep pattern and subsequent behaviour when awake are considered normal by both the parent or guardian and the Accident and Emergency staff. This is discussed further in Section 4.5.

Deterioration

Change in the level of consciousness is even more important than its absolute level on arrival in the A and E department. Frequent assessment of conscious level is therefore necessary, the interval between examination being dictated by the clinical state. Initially this may be as frequent as every five minutes in patients with impaired consciousness. Those patients who are fully conscious with an EMV of 4,6,5 should be reassessed within half an hour and certainly before contemplating discharge (Table 5.2; Section 5.3).

Patients occasionally deteriorate shortly after an initial assessment has suggested that they are fully conscious and have been minimally injured. In retrospect, the initial examination might have been too cursory and important clues might have been overlooked. For example, the complaint of severe headache or an unusually long post-traumatic amnesia. More commonly the patient might have been assumed to have been fully conscious whereas there was slight impairment of higher intellectual function (Section 4.2). It is important to have a challenging conversation with the patient and not merely to exchange platitudes. It is remarkable how people can convey the impression of normal mentation when they are merely responding in a random manner by the use of well-known phrases to a series of trivial questions. In the case of children it is extremely important to consider the opinion of the parents. They are usually more able to assess change in conscious level than is the examining doctor or nurse.

Patients who have significant 'primary brain injury' are usually unconscious from the outset and their assessment and management is outside the scope of this text. Deterioration due to so-called 'secondary brain injury' is usually due to hypoxia and/or hypercarbia raising intracranial pressure. Systemic injury causing hypovolaemic shock and chest injury causing hypoxaemia should also be considered. The most important neurosurgical consideration is the possible development of an extradural haematoma (Section 4.2).

Non-traumatic causes of deterioration in conscious level may be directly or coincidentally associated with a minor head injury. For example, the patient might have been involved in an accident because of the development of hypoglycaemia. The initial response to the injury would be to produce a transient hyperglycaemia. This might allow some improvement in conscious level followed by a deterioration in the A and E department (Section 4.2). Patients who are inebriated or under the influence of medication or illegal drugs are unlikely to deteriorate in the A and E department from that cause. However, an epileptic might have a second attack within the department and if his airway is not clearly secured the resultant hypoxia may cause a deterioration in the level of consciousness.

Deterioration due to non-traumatic causes and to cardiorespiratory incompetence is important and must be excluded. However, it is wise to assume that a patient who is walking and talking on arrival in the A and E department and who then deteriorates is also at risk from the development of an expanding intracranial haematoma. The length of time to diagnosis and treatment of this condition is directly related to the long-term prognosis [5].

2.7 LONG TRACT SIGNS

The initial assessment referred to at the beginning of this chapter should detect any gross limb asymmetry. A more specific examination of the limbs is only required in those fully conscious patients who have an abnormal gait or leg agility, or who are unable to maintain outstretched, upturned arms with their eyes closed. In such patients and in all those who have an impaired level of consciousness, formal testing of limb movements and an assessment of power, sensation and reflexes must be undertaken.

Occasionally a depressed skull fracture may produce discrete focal signs reflected in abnormal limb function, without loss of consciousness. This possibility will usually have been drawn to the examiner's attention by features in the history (e.g. method of wounding) or by scalp examination. However, the great majority of patients with abnormal long tract signs also exhibit a depression in level of consciousness.

2.8 THE EYES

Pupil reaction

This should be tested in a dark room using a bright light. A crisp pupil response is best elicited by switching on the torch when it is already positioned in front of the eye. Drawing the illuminated torch across the visual field increases the incident light more gradually and therefore the pupil response may not be as brisk. Ideally the switch on the torch should have a silent operation as a click may startle the patient and thereby cause reflex constriction through a non-visual reflex.

The consensual light reflex is valuable only if there is no response to the direct test. The pathways involved in these reflexes are described in Fig. 2.7.

Pupil reaction is more important than pupil size. If both pupils react to light briskly and the patient is fully conscious, any inequality of size usually represents a chronic problem or a normal variant. However, any change in pupil response should be assumed to reflect an increase in the intracranial pressure and the patient treated appropriately (Section 4.2). It must be emphasized that this is usually a late sign of rising pressure causing compression of the 3rd nerve and that changes in the level of consciousness are much more sensitive and early indicants of deterioration. This is represented diagramatically in figure 5.2.

Patients with a solitary unreactive pupil who are otherwise neurologically intact have usually suffered direct trauma to the eye – or have a prosthesis!

If a patient has an apparently inappropriate pupil size or response when contrasted with the general neurological examination,

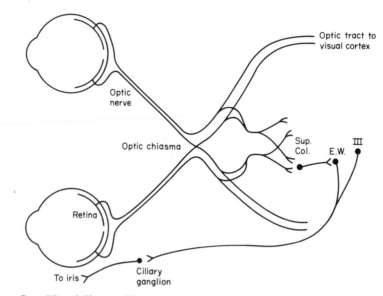

Fig. 2.7 The light reflex: The different fibres leave the optic tract just before the geniculate body and end in the superior colliculus. An internuncial neurone connects this to the Edinger Westphal nucleus of the occulomotor nerve which terminates at the ciliary ganglion. This pathway receives less collateral fibres than ipsilateral afferents. The consensual light reflex is therefore weaker than the direct light reflex.

consider the effects of any drugs which may have been given systemically or locally. Examples include the miotic effect of narcotic analgesics and the cycloplegic effects of homatropine which might have been given unwisely by a colleague to enhance fundoscopy.

Visual field

Examination of the visual field can be quickly carried out in the co-operative patient by confrontation and 'eye-balling'. Each eye is tested in turn, using the examiner's extended and intermittently moving hands to compare the examiner's peripheral vision with that of the patient.

Fundoscopy

This should be carried out routinely without the aid of cycloplegic drugs. The objectives of this examination are to exclude local damage to the retina and to assess the optic disc. In infants the finding of retinal haemorrhages is almost diagnostic of a 'shaking injury' and child abuse should be suspected.

Bilateral papilloedema is usually produced by a gradual rise in intracranial pressure over some days or weeks, such as may occur with a chronic subdural haematoma. Papilloedema is unlikely to be detected within a few hours of acute head injury even when this is associated with a rise in intracranial pressure in the unconscious patient.

Eye movements

These are tested using an an illuminated torch. The patient should be asked if he sees double at any stage during this test. Oculomotor (3rd nerve) palsy is usually associated with an injury of sufficient severity to cause loss of consciousness (Section 4.2). The affected eye gazes laterally and downwards. The pupil is dilated and unresponsive to light. There may be a ptosis. If the patient is conscious he will report diplopia on upward and inward gaze.

Abducent (6th nerve) palsy may be caused by the compressive effects of an intracranial haematoma. Alternatively the nerve may be damaged by a fracture of the petrous temporal bone. Occasionally it occurs in an otherwise uncomplicated minor head injury. There is diplopia on attempted lateral gaze (Fig. 2.8).

The trochlea (4th) nerve may be damaged at the same time as the 3rd or 6th or by fractures involving the orbit or cavernous sinus. Isolated lesions of this nerve are rare although damage to the superior oblique muscle and its pulley system can occur as a consequence of injury to the orbit. Impairment of function causes inability to turn the affected eye downwards and outwards.

Nystagmus

A rhythmical jerking of the eye on lateral gazing may occur spontaneously in the head injured patient or may be initiated on testing eye movements or changing the position of the head (Fig. 2.9). It is usually associated with damage to the vestibulo–cochlear apparatus which may complicate a fracture of the petrous temporal bone. The

(a)

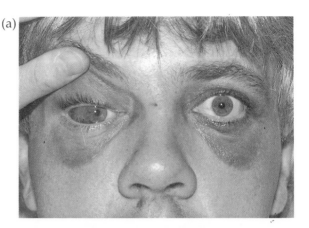

(b)

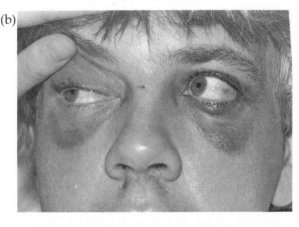

(c)

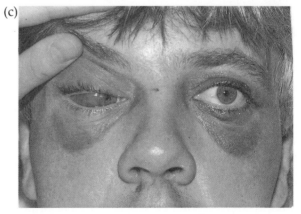

Fig. 2.8 Left abducent palsy and frontal fracture with bilateral peri-orbital haematoma: (a) looking forwards; (b) looking to the right; (c) looking to the left.

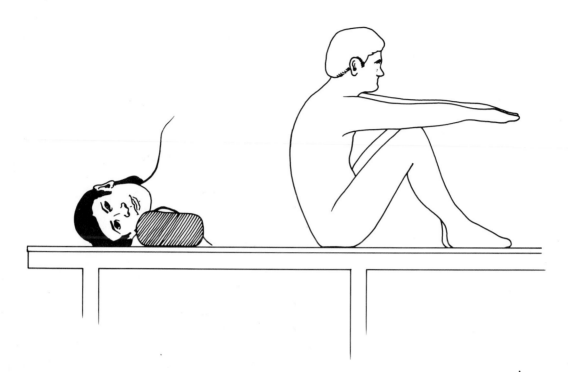

Fig. 2.9 Test for positional vertigo and nystagmus. First ensure that the patient does not have a spinal problem. Then ask him to sit on the couch. Hold his head, turned towards you, and gently lower it until it is about 45° below horizontal, with the large pillow under the patient's chest. This manoeuvre should take about 3 s and should be maintained for 20 s – or less if nystagmus or vertigo are evident. The procedure should be repeated with the head turned to the opposite side.

conscious patient complains of vertigo and nausea and may vomit. The nystagmus may have been present before the head injury and one of its many causes, alcohol abuse, may have precipitated the accident.

Visual acuity

Ideally this should be tested using a Snellen's chart [6] at six metres, but a test of near vision with a reduced Snellen's chart or newspaper print will usually suffice (Fig. 2.10). For young children who cannot read letters, the Kay Picture Test [7] provides a suitable alternative.

Swelling and bruising may cause the eyelids to close within a few hours of injury. If this has occurred by the time the patient presents to the department it is worthwhile recording whether light can be detected through the closed lids. An attempt should be made to open the lids gently and slowly and this can often be achieved by gentle pressure which dissipates some of the periorbital swelling. This initial examination, which may be facilitated by the application of amethocaine eyedrops, is also used to assess pupil size and response and to detect any local damage.

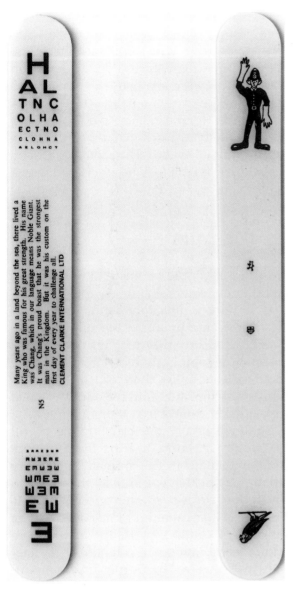

Fig. 2.10 Reduced Snellen's chart: to be used at about 33 cm to test visual acuity. Remember to allow patient to wear 'reading glasses' if available (Clement Clarke International Ltd).

Cornea

Corneal examination is aided by the use of a hand lens or the ophthalmoscope adjusted to +20. Irregularity of the pupil, a 'softness' of the anterior chamber, or the presence of blood in the anterior chamber (hyphaema), indicates the presence of a significant intra-ocular injury. Management is discussed in Section 4.4

Optic nerve

Direct damage to the optic nerve may be caused by fracture at the base of the skull or penetration of the orbit. This will result in partial or complete loss of vision and hence an absent direct pupillary response. However, the crossed consensual light reflex will be present (see Fig. 2.7). The optic nerve is also threatened by an expanding retrobulbar haemorrhage. This may present as a proptosis (Section 1.4).

Orbit

A blow-out fracture of the orbit can occur in combination with other 'mid-face' fractures but may be an isolated injury – for example caused by a squash ball. There may be remarkably little intraocular damage or evident external injury to the periorbital tissues. The globe itself is more resilient than the thin floor of the orbit, so a direct blow to the eye may cause herniation of the orbital contents down into the maxillary antrum or, less commonly, medial herniation into the ethmoidal sinus. Check for diplopia, a painful restriction of extraocular movements and 'globe retraction' on

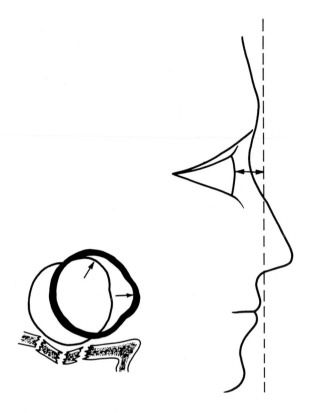

Fig. 2.11 Globe retraction test. The edge of a card, represented by the dashed line, is held against the eyebrow and upper lip. The distance between the card and the globe is increased on upward gaze by a 'blow-out' fracture of the orbital floor which prevents normal globe rotation (thin outline in inset figure).

attempted upward gaze (Fig 2.11). Once periorbital swelling has resolved, enophthalmos and lowering of the pupillary level may be apparent.

Frontal fossa

A fracture of the frontal fossa typically produces periorbital haematoma(ta) with purple discoloration limited to the orbital margin(s) within a few hours. The association of subconjunctival haemorrhage without a posterior limit and nasal bleeding are confirmatory features (Fig. 2.12). When these features are bilateral, the appearance resembles the eyes of a panda (Fig. 2.13). A blow to the forehead may produce a nontender unilateral black eye, quickly involving the upper eyelid. This denotes a deep scalp bruise which may be associated with a skull fracture (Fig. 2.14).

2.9 THE EARS

No attempt should be made to remove any blood in the external auditory meatus. This may introduce infection, as may the introduction of an auroscope. Bleeding into the external auditory meatus after head injury is usually a complication of a fracture of the middle cranial fossa, therefore the introduction of any infection into the auditory canal may quickly extend into the brain.

If there is no obvious bleeding it is useful to conduct a simple hearing test (whisper from one metre). The human voice or a ticking wristwatch will suffice. If damage to the middle ear is suspected and no blood is present in the canal an auroscope may be introduced cautiously. Injury to the tympanic membrane or evidence of a haemotympanum (a dark purple appearance of the drum) may be detected. Although this may be due to local trauma it is wise to assume that there is a fracture of the middle cranial fossa (Section 4.2). A late sign of this fracture is bruising over the mastoid region (Battle's sign, Fig. 2.15) but this may take more than 24 hours to develop.

The conscious patient who becomes unsteady when asked to stand with eyes

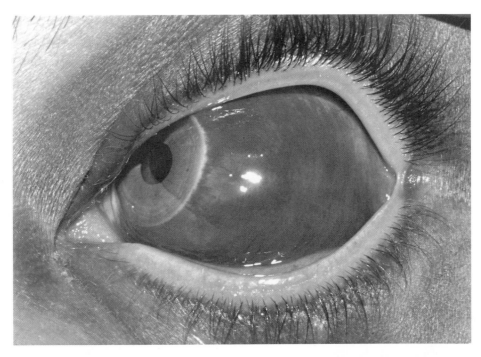

Fig. 2.12 Frontal fracture producing subconjunctival haemorrhage.

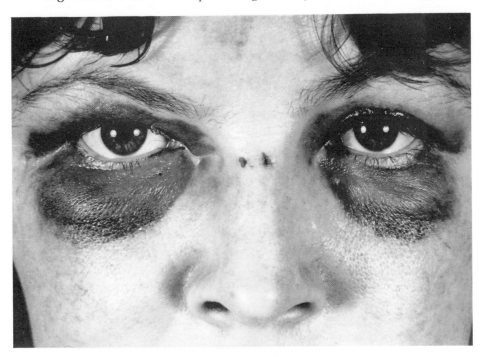

Fig. 2.13 Panda eyes.

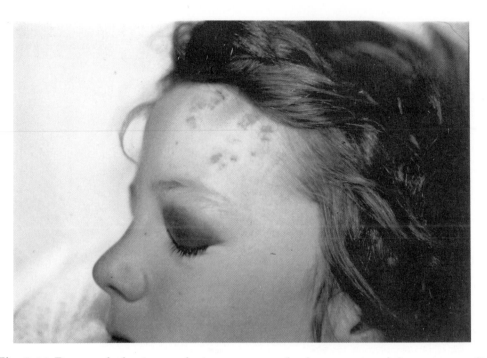

Fig. 2.14 Deep scalp bruise producing a non-tender haematoma of the upper eyelid.

closed and feet together is exhibiting a positive Romberg's sign. This may be due to labyrinthine damage.

2.10 OTHER CRANIAL NERVES

Cranial nerve (i)

Anosmia usually results from damage to the olfactory nerves by a deceleration force as they pass through the base of the skull at the cribriform plate. The condition is much more common than is generally recognized. A bar of hospital soap is all that is required to test the presence of olfaction. Clearly patients whose noses are blocked with blood cannot be accurately tested. A repeat examination will be necessary at a later date.

Cranial nerve (v)

Injury to the trigeminal nerve is commonly associated with facial fractures. Facial sensation is tested on both sides at the same time but local facial swelling may modify appreciation of sensation. The supra-orbital nerve (v(a)) may be damaged by a frontal fracture. Anaesthesia can extend back onto the vertex, at least 15 cm behind the eyebrows. This nerve may also be injured by simple laceration of the forehead. The infra-orbital nerve (v(b)) may be injured in the infra-orbital canal by malar or maxillary fractures. Numbness extends to the upper lip, upper incisors and the side of the nose. Mandibular fracture may damage the mental nerve (v(c)) causing anaesthesia of the lower lip and gum.

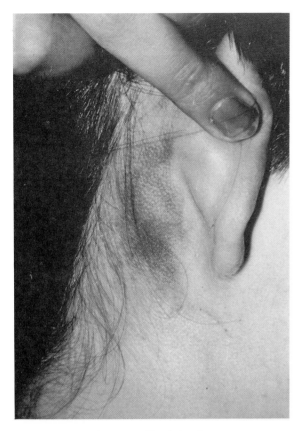

Fig. 2.15 Battle's sign.

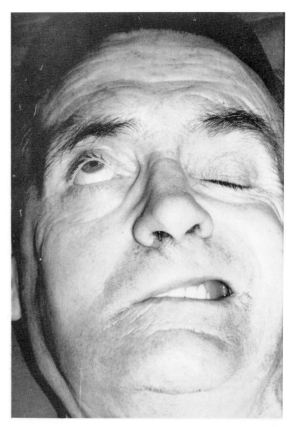

Fig. 2.16 Right lower motor neurone facial palsy with protective upward rotation of the globe.

Cranial nerve (vii)

Facial weakness may be associated with fracture of the petrous temporal bone. This is a lower motor neurone palsy involving the whole of one side of the face (Fig. 2.16). Its early recognition and documentation is valuable in assessing prognosis (Section 6.2).

An upper motor neurone facial weakness may be caused by damage to the contralateral cerebral hemisphere. Classically this spares the frontalis muscle and in the context of head injury is usually associated with long tract signs in the arms or legs.

There may also be a speech deficit if the injury is to the dominant hemisphere.

Cranial nerves (ix), (x), (xi), (xii)

These cranial nerves can be tested quickly by asking the patient to say 'Aaah' ((ix) and (x) nerves), to put out the tongue ((xii) nerve) and to shrug the shoulders ((xi) nerve). The tongue and gums can be examined whilst the mouth is open – the former for evidence of injury and the latter

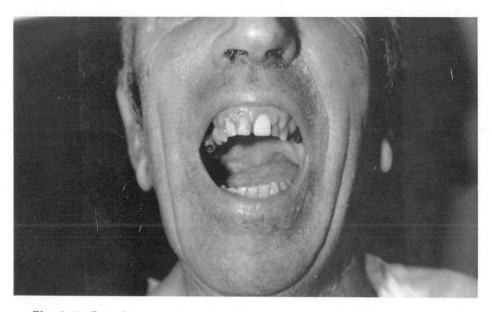

Fig. 2.17 Gum hypertrophy caused by Phenytoin anticonvulsant therapy.

for hypertrophy caused by Phenytoin anticonvulsant therapy (Fig. 2.17).

Although it is unusual for a patient with a minor head injury to exhibit abnormalities in these nerves, specific damage to them may be inflicted by stab wounds of the neck or by damage inflicted by intra-oral foreign bodies (e.g. impaling on a knitting needle).

2.11 THE EXTENT OF THE NEUROLOGICAL EXAMINATION

Patients with evident brain injury and specific neurological signs clearly demand careful neurological assessment and detailed documentation. Conversely it might be thought unnecessary to record the many negative findings in a neurological assessment of a patient with an apparently minor head injury. Indeed it is tempting to question the value of a full assessment of the central nervous system in such patients. Clearly it must not be carried out before immediate resuscitation of the patient and the assessment and management of reversible conditions relating to the cardiorespiratory system. Subsequently a compromise must be reached between the ideal comprehensive neurological assessment, which is time-consuming, and a cursory glance which might overlook important components of the injury.

Tables 2.2 and 2.3 present a method of assessment and documentation which could be adopted by casualty officers who are hard-pressed for time but wish to pick up all the important neurological findings. The positive and negative findings thereby recorded may be of immediate value when considering neurosurgical referral and also, at a later date, for research purposes or as the basis for court evidence.

Table 2.2 Example of 'History Stamp'

Time of injury ....   Time of examination ....

Alcohol:	No	Yes			
PTA (min):	No	Yes	< 5	5–60	> 60

Symptoms: No   Yes   Headache ⟨ Severe / Mild

Nausea   Vomiting   Dizziness   Visual
Other ....

Past medical history:

Drugs:

Table 2.3 Example of 'Examination stamp'

Limb Mvts. Symmetrical:		Yes	No	
Pupils React:		Both	One	Neither
Equal:		Yes	No	

Cranial nerves (– intact; X – deficient; N – not examined)

Smell   ; Eye Mvts   ;   Visual fields   ;   Acuity   ;

Face ⟨ Sensation   ; / Motor   ;   Palate Mvt.   ;   Tongue Mvt.   ;

Hearing ⟨ Right   ; / Left   ;   Tymp. Memb. ⟨ Right / Left   ;   Fundoscopy   ;

Neck Mvt:	Full	Restricted	
G.C.S.:	Eyes	Motor	Verbal

Box 2

CASE HISTORY

A sixty-seven year old man was brought from an old people's home by ambulance. He had been seen to fall and strike the front of his head on a chair. He required assistance to walk and complained of an occipital headache. He was mildly confused but this had been his normal state for some years. Neck movement was painful. Limb movement was difficult to assess but his intrinsic hand movements were weak. He had a full bladder but normal peri-anal sensation.

X-rays of the skull, pelvis and hips showed no fracture. X-rays of the cervical spine showed marked spondylosis but no fracture.

What is the likely diagnosis?

In the elderly, a spinal cord injury is possible without a fracture or dislocation. This is termed the Central Cord Syndrome and occurs because the spinal cord is narrowed by cervical spondylosis and further reduced by extension of the neck and soft tissue injury. The initial management includes limiting the range of neck movement with a soft collar and catheterization of the bladder. With the help of physiotherapy good progress can be made in walking and bladder function although it is likely that there will be permanent mild hand stiffness.

Golden rules

'Normal' cervical spine X-rays do not exclude spinal cord injury.

3 Investigations

3.1 SYSTEMIC ASSESSMENT

It is essential to ensure the stability of the cardiorespiratory system before beginning a specific investigation of cerebral function. This is achieved by carrying out a quick general examination followed by measurement of pulse, blood pressure, respiratory rate and, where appropriate, the arterial blood gases.

Assuming that there are no major extracranial problems, a rising blood pressure and falling pulse rate are indicative of increasing intracranial pressure. However, these are very late signs and have always been preceded by other indications of raised

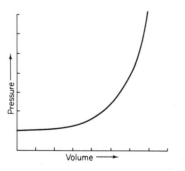

Fig. 3.1 Relationship between intracranial pressure and volume.

intracranial pressure. Indeed significant brain swelling can occur with minimal increase in intracranial pressure (Fig. 3.1.) Deterioration in level of consciousness and responsiveness followed by changes in pupil reaction are more relevant indicators to be used in the A and E department.

3.2 SKULL X-RAY

Skull radiography is not only an important discriminator in a patient with an apparently minor head injury who might otherwise be discharged, but is also relevant in planning proper care for the admitted patient. Clearly it is not the most important investigation in the multiply injured patient. However, failure to detect a skull fracture may influence priorities in management and delay prophylactic antibiotic therapy. The incidence of intracranial haematoma is 400 times higher in patients who have vault fractures than in those who do not.

Accident and Emergency departments are often criticized for requesting too many skull radiographs. It is inevitable that many 'negative' films will have been requested, but the knowledge that there is no skull vault fracture is important as it will often allow the clinician to discharge home the patient with a minor head injury. However in order to reduce unnecessary demands on the radiology service it is essential to develop guidelines which allow optimal use of skull radiography. These should balance the expense of the investigation against the savings to be made by confidently discharging patients who are very unlikely to develop complications. In 1987 the cost of a skull radiograph series was £25 compared with £125 for a 24 hour period of hospital observation.

Indications for skull radiography include:

- The patient does not have a consecutive memory of events since the accident. This includes patients who give a vague or implausible account of events.

- Any suggestion of epileptic fits.

- When the head injury is sustained at considerable speed (for example all road traffic accidents and falling from more than two metres).

- Impact injuries sustained to the temporal area of the scalp.

- Open scalp wounds unless demonstrably superficial.

- Whenever the injuring agent is known to be heavy or hard irrespective of scalp contact site.

- Patients with abnormal neurological signs or depressed conscious level.

- Patient who have vomited within the past 12 hours or complain of persistent generalized headache. (It will usually be found that these patients have also fulfilled one or more of the above indications for skull radiography.)

Skull radiography is unnecessary if the patient has sustained a witnessed occipital, parietal or frontal injury at low speed against a relatively soft, flat surface with no loss of consciousness and, on initial examination, no neurological abnormalities. Similarly those who have only sustained superficial clean scalp lacerations in low speed accidents and superficial incised wounds caused by a knife do not merit X-ray. Examples include someone who falls forwards onto a carpet and presents with a frontal haematoma but has not been knocked out and is normal on presentation to the A and E department, and someone who sustains a scalp laceration by catching his head on barbed wire.

Standard views

These must include a 'brow-up' lateral film of the injured side (both sides if in any doubt), an anteroposterior (AP) film, and a 30° 'Towne's' view (Fig. 3.2). The quality of the films must be good if skull fractures are to be detected. Inevitably some films will be of poor quality if the patient is uncooperative. Examples of unacceptable films are given in Fig. 3.3. Fractures cannot be excluded on such films.

Each film should be examined on a standard viewing box fitted with a spotlight. A magnifying glass is very helpful in the interpretation of abnormalities. The lateral film shows the side nearest to the plate in sharper focus (i.e. the left parietal and temporal regions in a left lateral film). The anteroposterior film is used to assess the frontal region and the Towne's view is ideal for the occipital bone. All these films can be taken with the patient supine and without undue neck movement (Fig. 3.4).

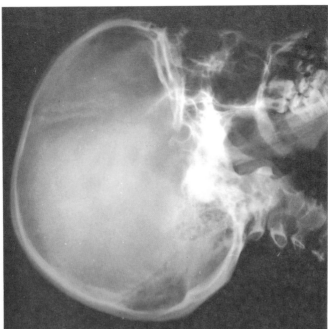

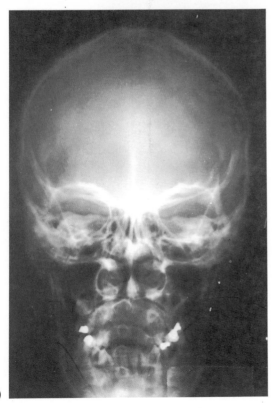

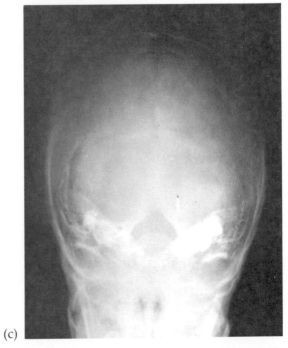

Fig. 3.2 Standard radiological view of the skull: (a) brow-up lateral; (b) anteroposterior; (c) Townes (AP 30°).

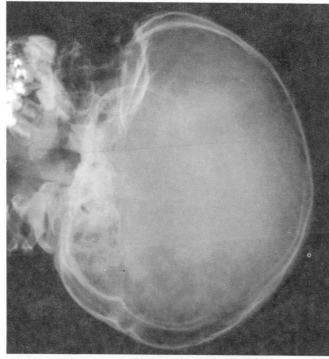

(a)

Fig. 3.3 Examples of poor quality skull radiographs: (a) brow-up lateral – the rotated view may be falsely interpreted as showing an occipital depressed fracture; (b) anteroposterior – the supraorbital region is not clearly seen due to superimposition of the petrous temporal complex; (c) Townes – a low occipital fracture may be obscured by the petrous temporal complex.

Fig. 3.4 (*opposite*) Patient and tube positions for skull radiography: (a) brow-up lateral; (b) anteroposterior; (c) Townes.

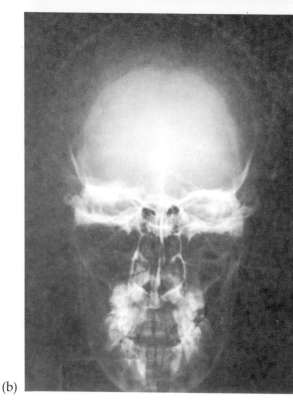

(b)

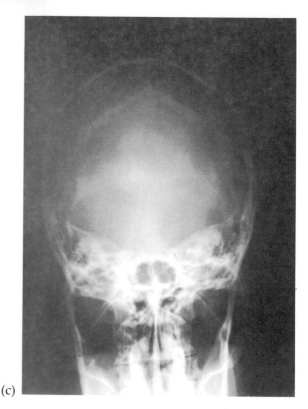

(c)

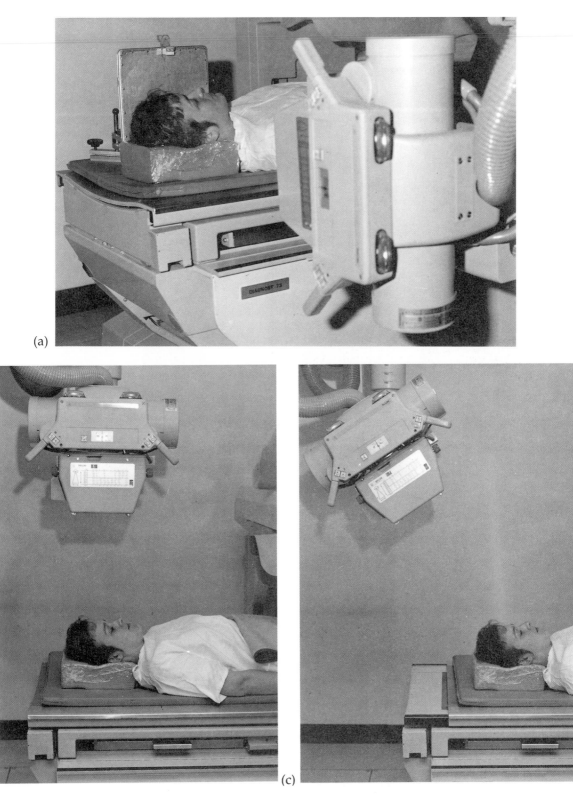

(a)

(b)

(c)

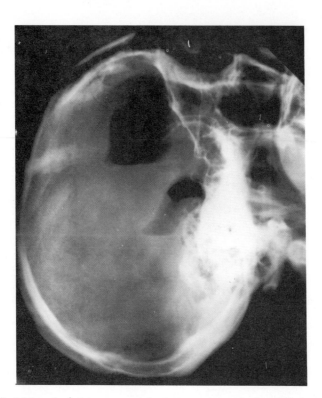

Fig. 3.5 Fluid level and intracranial air in a severely head injured patient.

Intracranial air, introduced via a fracture in the base of the skull or an air sinus, is more likely to be demonstrated on a 'brow-up' lateral film. Likewise fluid levels may be evident (Fig. 3.5). It may not be possible to obtain this view in an uncooperative patient. In this case it may be necessary to turn the patient's head through 90° so that the ear rests on a horizontal plane. Intracranial air or fluid may not appear on this 'turned lateral' view (Fig. 3.6).

Other views

Other views of the skull which are frequently useful in the A and E department are tangential and posteroanterior (PA). The latter may be necessary to demonstrate clearly the supraorbital region (Fig. 3.7) and the former to identify and determine the extent of a depressed fracture (see Fig. 3.13). Foreign bodies such as glass fragments will show up best on 'soft tissue' radiographs (Fig. 3.8).

Radiological confirmation of basal skull fracture is difficult and should not be sought by taking special views. The clinical diagnosis is usually self-evident. A view of the base of the skull is radiologically possible but requires considerable hyper-extension of the cervical spine. This is very dangerous in recently head injured patients who may have a neck injury.

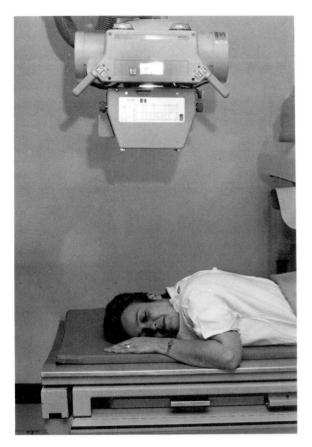

Fig. 3.6 Patient and tube position for the 'turned-lateral' view.

Films should never be examined without first looking carefully at the patient and the scalp. Knowledge of the direction and severity of the injury together with local scalp damage will help to highlight the importance of examination of certain parts of the films.

Linear fractures

Crisp and sharp lines of measurable finite length usually represent linear fractures (Fig. 3.9). Although soft tissue healing and

adequate repair occurs at the site of a linear vault fracture, radiological evidence of bone union is usually delayed in adults, sometimes for years. The early periosteal response at the site of long bone fractures is not seen in the skull. However softening of the fracture line with bridging is commonly seen after some months and in children fractures usually disappear within six months.

Widening of the suture line by more than 2 mm between two vault bones – a feature called diastasis – is seen particularly in head injured children. The diagnosis can usually be made by comparing the width of the irregular lucent area with the appearance on the undamaged side. These injuries should be treated similarly to linear vault fractures.

Depression of the skull vault

This is always associated with local scalp injury (it may be deceptively small, but will be present). The fracture may be evident on the standard views. Classically there is an area of increased lucency, due to separation of the bones, and another area of increased density due to overlapping. The displaced bony fragments often appear as a double density – inner and outer skull tables being viewed tangentially (Figs 3.10 and 3.11). When the depressed fracture is caused by a blunt instrument such as a hammer there is a characteristic circular lucency within which opaque lines radiate like the spokes of a wheel (Fig. 3.12). The extent of the depression is best demonstrated by a view taken tangential to the point of impact (Fig. 3.13). Such injuries are not necessarily associated with loss of consciousness. The patient may well present as a 'minor head injury'.

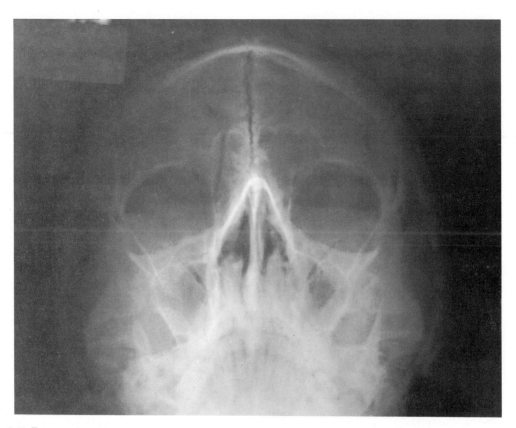

Fig. 3.7 Posteroanterior view showing right frontal fracture and coincidental metopic suture.

Vascular markings and suture lines

These are sometimes confused with fracture lines. Knowledge of the position of suture lines and the characteristics of vascular markings (Fig. 3.14) usually enables them to be excluded. Vascular markings produced by meningeal vessels have a wide curvilinear and branching appearance. It is usually difficult to identify their termination and origin and they are of variable density. On the lateral view vascular markings tend to radiate upwards from the base of the skull from the region of the soft tissue marking of the pinna. Markings at right angles to these vessels should be considered to represent fractures.

Common normal variants

Normal anatomical variants which mimic skull fracture are described in Table 3.1 and shown in Figs 3.15–3.17. Beware the metopic suture which is present in young children and persists in up to 10% of the adult population, and wormian bones occurring along the lines of the sutures. Venous lacunae, particularly in relation to the superior saggital sinus, may have one crisp

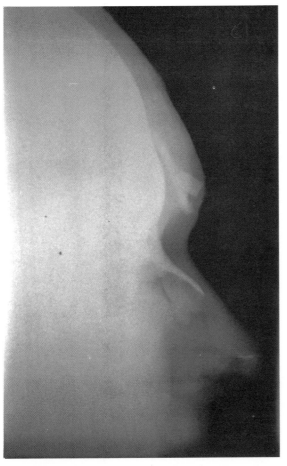

Fig. 3.8 Soft tissue radiograph showing windscreen glass.

margin but not the crescentic increased density characteristic of a depressed fracture.

The pineal gland is a midline structure which is calcified with increasing age. It can then be identified on the lateral view and its lateral displacement assessed on the AP and Towne's views. The choroid plexuses may be calcified but their position is variable in the normal brain and therefore apparent asymmetry cannot be used to indicate brain shift.

X-ray audit

A rapid, reliable and consistent method of reporting the radiologist's comments on A and E skull radiographs must be established. The clinician's findings must be made available to the radiologist and should at least indicate the site of injury. Ideally the radiologist's report should accompany the films back to the casualty officer but this is rarely possible outside office hours. Therefore an efficient patient recall system is essential if the occasional false negative diagnoses of the casualty officer are to be quickly detected and corrected.

3.3 OTHER X-RAYS

Facial X-rays

The facial skeleton is built to withstand the compressive forces of mastication but not the advancing fist or boot. The crumbling of the facial skeleton in response to such an anteroposterior force absorbs much of its energy and may protect the brain somewhat from the full effects of the insult.

However, injury to the face is commonly associated with brain injury in victims of assault and in those vehicle occupants who have not been restrained by a safety belt. The clinical examination of the face is described in Section 2.5 and will determine the need for facial radiographs. Remember that 'skull X-rays' will not show clearly nasal or other facial bones and to avoid unnecessary radiographs the precise area of interest must be indicated to the radiographer

Cervical spine X-rays

In contrast to serious facial injury, damage to the cervical spine may be occult. Many

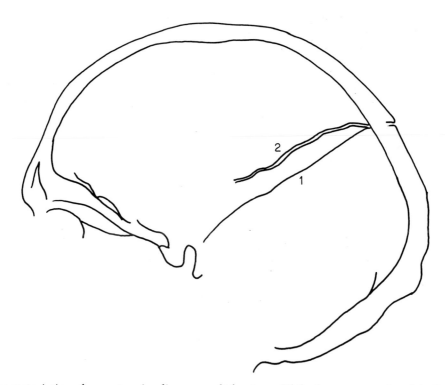

Fig. 3.9 Characteristics of an extensive linear vault fracture. This shows as a crisp thin line (1) on the side of the skull adjacent to the X-ray film, but as a wide hazy line (2) on the opposite side of the skull.

head injuries are sustained by the relatively mobile head hitting a fixed object, e.g in a road traffic accident or a fall from a height. Where considerable force is applied across the cervical spine, the patient's symptoms may initially be due to the injuries to scalp and brain but not to the neck (Section 1.3). Radiographs of the cervical spine should always be taken in these circumstances and if the patient is confused or distracted by other painful injuries (Section 2.3). In contrast, when a mobile object strikes the stationary head, but does not have sufficient energy to set the head in motion, there will be little effect on the cervical spine and radiographs are usually not required.

The lateral view is the most important.

Damage to the vertebral column is particularly common at the junctions of mobile and fixed sections, e.g. at C7/T1. It is essential that all seven cervical vertebrae are visualized. To achieve this it may be necessary to pull the arms down whilst the film is being taken. Failure to visualize C7 should be discussed with a radiologist as it may be necessary to proceed to tomography or CT scan if there is the slightest suspicion of a neck injury. The other standard cervical spine views are the anteroposterior for C2–C7 and the coned view through the open mouth for C1 and the odontoid peg.

Alignment of the cervical vertebrae is best assessed on a lateral view. There should be a slight posterior-facing concavity

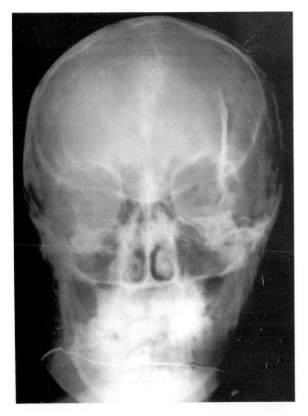

Fig. 3.10 AP view of depressed fracture of left frontal bone showing characteristic double density.

(lordosis) described by the posterior borders of the vertebral bodies. Slight laxity at C2/3, particularly in children, is normal (Fig. 3.18). The alignment of each apophyseal joint should be checked and the continuity of the spinous processes confirmed. The soft tissue shadow in front of the anterior border of the vertebral bodies, representing the posterior pharyngeal musculature, may be increased by haematoma and tissue oedema. The normal width of this 'posterior pharyngeal space' is between 1.5 mm and 4.5 mm at C3 level. At the level of C6 the 'post-tracheal space' measures between

8 mm and 18 mm, i.e. less than the width of that vertebral body. Any increase should be considered to be due to haematoma associated with ligament and/or bony injury. More rarely it is associated with direct damage to the pharynx.

3.4 OTHER INVESTIGATIONS

Echo encephalography

The former use of ultrasound equipment to detect displacement of the falx required careful application by skilled clinicians with some medical physics training. The advent of computerized tomography and the unreliable results of ultrasound obtained in unskilled hands led to the gradual disappearance of these relatively cheap machines from Accident and Emergency departments. However, the development of the automatic midline computer and the replacement of the A mode by the Grey scale display both allow accurate assessment of midline structures in a more reproducible form. Unfortunately, the clinician's disappointment with the earlier A mode machines has led to reluctance to use these more reliable 'midliners'. Although they are probably superfluous in departments which have early access to CT scanning facilities they could fulfil a useful role in district general hospitals and smaller units without such equipment. The skull vault prevents the use of Grey scale diagnostic ultrasound to visualize intracranial structures over the age of six months but in neonates and infants examination via the open fontanelles can reveal useful information. The technique is now used extensively in special care baby units and can be applied to head injury in infants.

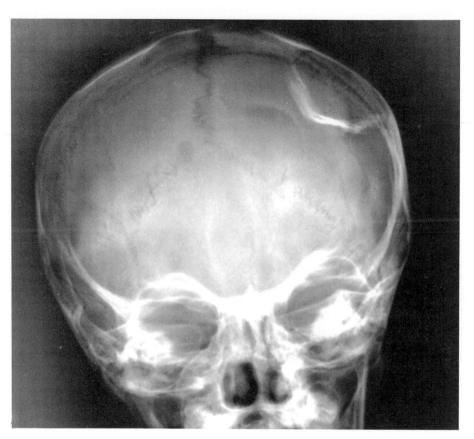

Fig. 3.11 AP view of depressed vault fracture.

Computed tomography

The development of this investigation has revolutionized the assessment and management of head injured patients. Columnated and fan-shaped beams of X-rays scan the brain in a series of tomographic cuts 15 mm thick. Each slice is traversed linearly by the X-ray source and detectors (rather than in an arc as in conventional tomography) and then repeated every 10° until a 180° examination has been completed. The absorption coefficient of each X-ray photon is computed to build up a two-dimensional picture of the scanned area which reflects depth of tissue as well as its density and surface projection.

Vault and basal fractures can be identified on CT scan but this is not generally considered to be a reason for abandoning plain radiography. At 1987 prices a plain skull series costs about £25 whereas a CT scan of the brain costs £95. More importantly the capacity of most scanning units would be overwhelmed were all head injured patients to be routinely scanned *ab initio*. Out of office hours at least 30 minutes' preparatory work is required before the scanner is available for use. There is also the problem of obtaining expert radiological opinion to interpret the images obtained. For these

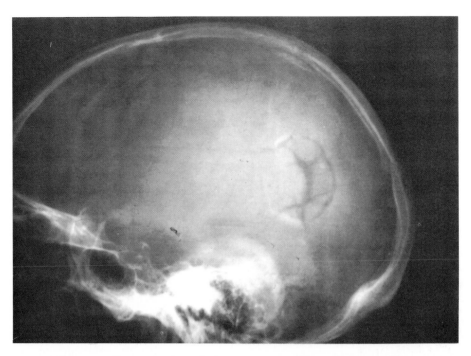

Fig. 3.12 Depressed vault fracture caused by a hammer blow.

reasons it is generally accepted that routine skull radiography is appropriate for the initial assessment of the head injured patient as indicated in the guidelines in section 3.2. Subsequent assessment by computerized tomography is generally determined after consultation between Accident and Emergency staff and the local neurosurgical service.

Although a few district general hospitals have scanners linked by telemetry to the regional neurosurgical service, this has not proved as popular or as valuable as initially expected. However, the increasing interest of neurosurgeons in the management of head injured patients and the wider distribution of CT scanners will inevitably lead to a more widespread use of this investigation in the early assessment of head injury at district general hospitals. It is to be hoped that the enthusiasm for CT scanning does not eclipse the need for basic clinical assessment of primary and potential secondary brain injury and the vigilance for extra-cranial pathology in the multiply injured patient.

NMR imaging

Nuclear magnetic resonance (NMR) spectroscopy measures the characteristic absorption and re-emission of energy by the hydrogen proton in a magnetic field. It is therefore quite unlike CT scanning which is a sophisticated form of radiological investigation. Contrasts of tone in the image represent variation in water content. For example, whereas the white rim of the periphery of the CT image represents bone,

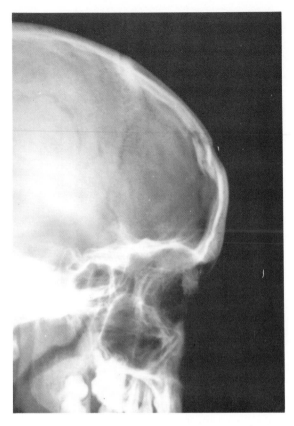

Fig. 3.13 Tangential view of a depressed vault fracture.

a rather similar appearance at the periphery of the NMR image represents marrow fat between the inner and outer tables of the skull. Although NMR imaging is in its clinical infancy it could have significant implications in the long term for the investigation of head injured patients. The distinction between white and grey matter is far superior to that obtained on CT scanning and areas of cerebral infarction and haemorrhage can be clearly identified. This suggests that NMR imaging will be particularly valuable in assessing the degree of primary brain injury after head trauma, in

contrast to CT scanning which cannot pick up areas of diffuse axonal injury and is more useful in recording the changes associated with secondary brain injury.

Biochemical markers

Serum levels of myelin basic protein, which is specific to the nervous system, have been shown to relate to severity of brain injury and to clinical outcome. The assay is not sufficiently sensitive to detect changes in patients with minor head injury and it is unclear at the present time if this failure to detect this biochemical marker in such cases is due to technical factors or its absence in the systemic circulation after relatively minor injury. Further investigation of this approach to the assessment of severity is warranted.

Percussion/auscultation of the skull

A novel approach to the detection of intracranial haematoma is the application of a stethoscope to the surface of the skull whilst percussing the centre of the forehead with a finger. The percussed note will not be heard as clearly when auscultation is carried out over an intracranial haematoma. It is claimed that systematic auscultation comparing the two sides of the vault from the frontal to the occipital regions will detect the majority of surface clots. Naturally the examination is not possible in areas of scalp haematoma. This method cannot be recommended as consistently reliable but may be of some value in isolated units which lack more sophisticated diagnostic tools.

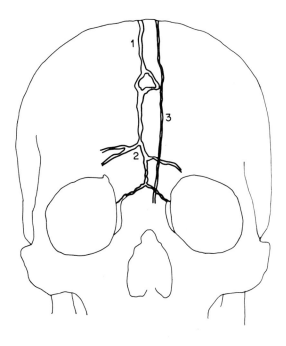

Fig. 3.14 Normal vascular markings and suture lines:

Fig. 3.14(a) AP view of child's skull. Note the persisting metopic suture in the frontal bone. This does not overlie the saggital suture because the radiograph has not been correctly centered. The division of the saggital suture into the two lambdoid sutures, at the lambda, is an imprecise feature in this particular skull. 1 = saggital suture, 2 = lambdoid suture, 3 = metopic suture.

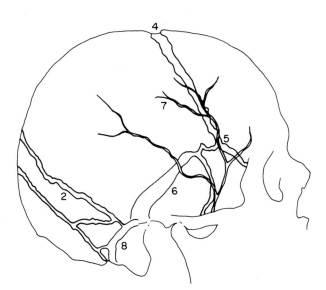

Fig. 3.14(b) Lateral view of child's skull. Note that sutures on both sides of the skull are seen on this projection. Whilst the bregma is often very thin, the lambda is thick and irregular. 2 = lambdoid suture, 4 = bregma (position of anterior fontanelle in infant), 5 = coronal suture, 6 = squamosal suture, 8 = Pinna.

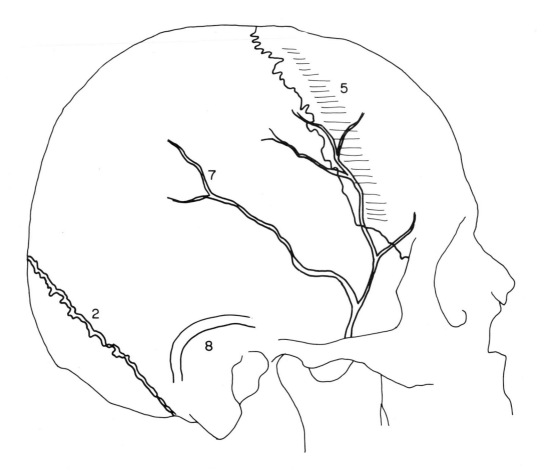

Fig. 3.14(c) Lateral view of adult's skull. The coronal and lambdoid sutures are fused but persist as wide irregular structures in contrast to the curvilinear branching radiolucencies produced by the meningeal vessels. Note the superoposterior radiation of the vessels. Darker lines at right angles in the region of the pterion (just in front of and above the pinna) usually represent undisplaced vault fractures. 2 = lambdoid suture, 5 = coronal suture, 7 = meningeal vessels, 8 = pinna.

Table 3.1 Normal anatomical variants (Numbers correspond with those in Figs 3.15, 3.16 and 3.17)

Neonate

Vault disproportionately larger in neonate than adult:

    Vault: Face in neonate 4:1

        Face in adult   3:2

Overlapping sutures may be seen in neonate secondary to moulding occurring during labour.

Scalp folds may mimic fracture line e.g. wrinkle in occiput

Child

Suture spreading is very common between the ages of 4 and 8.

1   Appearance and fusion of anterior fontanelle may mimic depressed fracture on lateral projection, but is clearly outlined on Townes view.

2   Wormian bones may be a normal variant in child and adult

3   Posterior part of squamosal suture may simulate a fracture

7   Metopic suture – may persist throughout life

8   Prominent nasofrontal suture may persist into adult life

10 Persistent membranous fissure simulating a fracture is commonest in infancy but may persist into adult life

11 Normal synchrondrosis between two parts of occipital bone in infant

Adult

4   Localized focal dural calcification

5   Focal calcification of falx cerebri

6   Calcification in the glomus of the choroid plexus of the lateral ventricle

9   Subsaggital suture of parietal bone

12 Overlapping of occipital bone (bathrocephaly) which may be confused with fracture

13 Midline occipital suture. This is also a common site for fracture!

15 Calcified pineal. Visible on lateral view in 50% of adults. Less frequently seen on AP view.

All ages

Matted hair, lacerations, clothing, hair bun, pillow may simulate a fracture. However the line may be seen to extend out past bone into the soft tissue shadow.

The upper part of the pinna (**14** in the figure) is often seen on the lateral projection.

Analysis of secretions

It is wise to assume that blood or serum escaping from the nose or ear after a head injury is mixed with cerebrospinal fluid, indicating a basal skull fracture. However confirmation is helpful and the fluid is often collected and sent for laboratory analysis. The usual request for biochemical analysis is of limited value because of the heavy contamination with blood. It is more logical to ask for a haemoglobin estimation. The finding of haemodilution when compared with systemic haemoglobin concentration

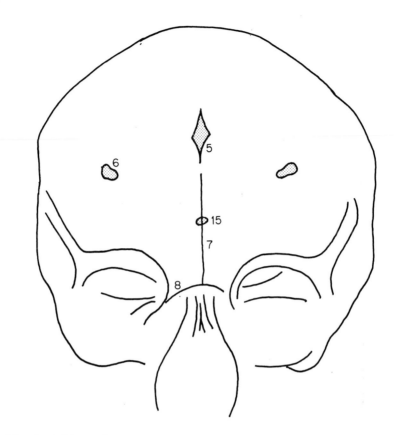

Fig. 3.15 Normal anatomical variants – AP view (see Table 3.1).

suggests the presence of cerebrospinal fluid in the secretion. Clear fluid leaking from the nose or ear can be analysed for sodium and chloride content and compared with normal serum electrolytes (Table 3.2). Testing for glucose is unreliable.

Blood alcohol concentration

There is a close linear relationship between blood and breath alcohol concentrations. Hand-held instruments which measure the latter are relatively inexpensive and quite accurate if used correctly and calibrated

regularly. It is important to entrain alveolar gases for analysis. This is relatively easy to achieve in conscious head injured patients but more difficult in the uncooperative or unconscious individual. Sampling nasal exhaled air in the latter may underestimate the blood alcohol concentration (BAC).

Knowledge of the blood alcohol concentration must not influence immediate management. It is however a valid investigation which can help to determine subsequent care, including rehabilitation. A high BAC must never be assumed to be the sole cause of a depressed level of consciousness and it is unusual for a level below 200 mg% to

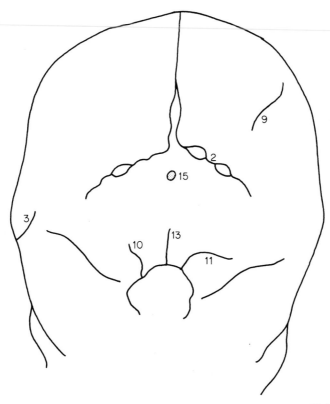

Fig. 3.16 Normal anatomical variants – Townes view (see Table 3.1).

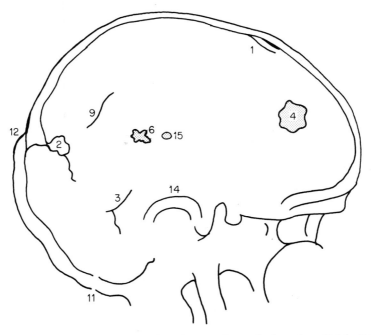

Fig. 3.17 Normal anatomical variants – lateral view (see Table 3.1).

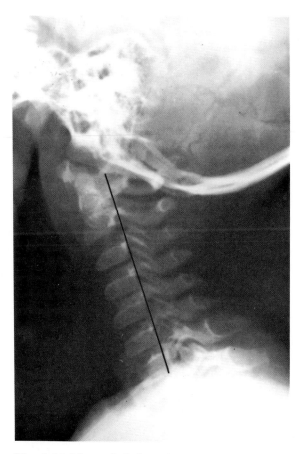

Fig. 3.18 Normal slight subluxation at C2/3 in a child.

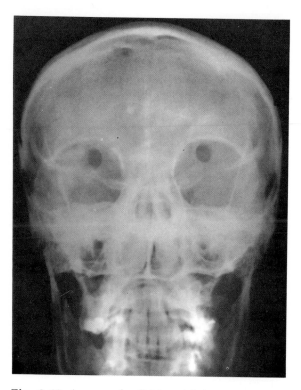

Fig. 3.19 A case of mild head injury (see Box 3 for details).

cause depression of the level of consciousness. Patients who are suspected of being chronic abusers of alcohol should have blood taken for a coagulation screen.

Photographs

Clinical photographs of scalp and facial injuries may be useful in subsequent legal proceedings. Plastic surgeons will find such records of value in recording the progress of treatment of complex facial wounds.

These photographs are to be considered the property of the Health Authority but should only be taken with consent of the patient.

Photographic records are also valuable in cases of suspected child abuse. These should be made by the in-patient team once the child has been admitted to hospital.

Table 3.2 Analysis of secretions

	CSF	Serum	Tears
	(mmol/l)		
Sodium	137–153	135–145	86–98
Chloride	119–131	95–105	112–130

3.5 INVESTIGATIONS TO AVOID IN A AND E

Intracranial pressure monitoring

Direct measurement of intracranial pressure by the placement of transducers either in the extradural or subarachnoid space is now generally practised in neurosurgical intensive care. Whilst of undoubted value in the longer term care of head injured patients, it can play no part in initial assessment and is therefore not considered an appropriate investigation to be carried out in the Accident and Emergency department.

Lumbar puncture

Any patient in whom the cause of neurological deterioration is in doubt and in whom lumbar puncture is indicated must be admitted. The investigation is not without risk in patients who may have raised intracranial pressure and it demands a sterile environment. The procedure may be undertaken in a high dependency unit, but not the A and E department.

Box 3

CASE HISTORY

A 35 year old man walks into the A and E department complaining of generalized vague headache three days after falling off his bicycle and sustaining a minor parietal graze. Clinical examination is unremarkable.

Comment on the radiograph (Fig. 3.19). What further action do you take?

The patient has had a previous operation for a meningioma via occipital burr holes. The pineal is displaced but the clinical picture is incompatible with the possibility of this being acute. Obtain and compare previous radiographs if possible.

Golden rule

Clinical assessment is more important than unsupported radiographs.

4 Treatment in the Accident and Emergency department

4.1 GENERAL RESUSCITATION

The initial management of the head injured patient is primarily directed to the rapid detection and treatment of life-threatening reversible conditions. These include obstruction of the airway, hypovolaemic shock due to occult haemorrhage, damage to the cervical spine and chest injury. Hypoglycaemic coma and opiate poisoning may be coincidental and should always be considered.

Any patient with the slightest reduction in conscious level should be assumed to have an impaired gag reflex. There is an increased incidence of nausea and vomiting after head injury, hence a risk of inhalation of vomitus. It is essential to remove dentures and clear the pharynx by suction prior to the insertion of an oral airway. The patient should be carefully turned to the lateral (recovery) position unless this is contraindicated by the presence of other injuries. If spinal or other major injuries preclude turning, endotracheal intubation should be considered. All trolleys used in the A and E department should be fitted with a mechanism which allows the patient to be placed in the 'head down tilt' position.

If there is little response to sucking out the pharynx (i.e patient has a significantly impaired gag reflex) endotracheal intubation should be performed. If the patient is restless and breathing spontaneously the help of a skilled anaesthetist should be sought. A clumsy attempt to introduce an endotracheal tube will cause a significant rise in intracranial pressure and may provoke cardiac dysrhythmias. Pre-oxygenation is essential. Correct placement of the tube is best confirmed by direct visualization of the vocal cords during its introduction. Subsequent assessment by checking breath sounds and chest movement is unreliable. If in any doubt disconnect the tube, leave it *in situ* and use a bag and mask over it rather than attempting immediate reinsertion. Flail chest and pneumothorax are potent causes of hypoxia and should be excluded by clinical examination and erect chest X-ray respectively.

Occult damage to the cervical spine must be considered at this stage (Section 2.3), but gentle movement of the neck is always acceptable in order to gain control of the airway. Early application of a firm cervical collar serves to limit undue neck movement and remind those who wish to move the patient of the possibility of an unstable cervical spine.

When the history suggests that the patient has been involved in an accident at high speed, has been brutally assaulted, or has fallen from a considerable height, it is reasonable to assume that there are multiple injuries. These may not be immediately evident and are not excluded by the finding of a normal blood pressure and pulse. In these circumstances, therefore, it is wise to establish venous access on the assumption that there is significant extracranial haemorrhage. Do not wait for the blood pressure to go down before putting up a drip. The presence of a head injury does not preclude adequate transfusion. Indeed any brain injury will be compounded by an inadequate cerebral circulation caused by systemic hypovolaemia or hypoxaemia. Urgent referral for appropriate in-patient care is essential in these cases.

4.2 PREVENTION OF SECONDARY BRAIN INJURY

Attention to the general resuscitative measures outlined above will do much to prevent unnecessary secondary brain injury (Table 4.1).

Airway and circulation

Hypoxia and, more importantly, hypercarbia and acidosis will cause an increase in intracranial pressure by a direct vasodilating effect on the cerebral microcirculation. Airway care must therefore be immaculate. The optimal arterial P_{CO_2} is between 25 and 30 mmHg. Cerebral autoregulation is impaired in injured brain areas and blood may be shunted from normal to damaged parts, compromising the supply to the former if the systemic pressure drops.

Infection

Contamination of compound scalp wounds may cause intracranial infection and abscess formation. Careful but thorough cleansing of such wounds is essential (Section 4.4). All clinically suspected fractures of the base of the skull should also be considered as compound injuries via the air sinuses or middle ear and therefore prone to infection. The early administration of intravenous antibiotics to patients with these injuries is essential. Flucloxacillin 500 mg (six hourly) for a compound vault fracture or a combination of Benzyl penicillin 600 mg and Sulphadimidine 1 g (six hourly) for a basal fracture are appropriate. The bleeding ear should be covered with a sterile pad.

Intracranial haematoma

The early detection of acute extradural haematoma is essential if the morbidity and

Table 4.1 Causes of secondary deterioration after head injury

- Airway obstruction causing hypercarbia
- Hypoxia
- Hypovolaemia
- Hypoglycaemia
- Extradural haemorrhage
- Brain swelling associated with raised intracranial pressure and focal brain damage
- Infection secondary to compound fracture of vault or base

mortality associated with this condition are to be minimized. The great majority of extradural haematoma in adults are complications of vault fractures, hence the importance of the selection criteria for skull radiography listed in Section 3.2. At all ages conscious level is the most important guide to prognosis. It is very rare for anyone who is fully conscious with normal mental acuity to suddenly deteriorate due to an intracranial haematoma. There is usually some initial alteration of behaviour or slowness of verbal response evident before disorientation develops. This can be difficult to assess in the young child, the elderly or the intoxicated patient.

The history of a varying level of consciousness following a trivial head injury sustained some days, or weeks, previously should alert the casualty officer to the possibility of a chronic subdural haematoma. This is particularly common in elderly patients. Recall of the accident may be poor, the relatives or warden dismissing the relevance of the minor injuries which are frequently sustained by such patients.

Clearly early neurosurgical advice should be sought on the further management of all these cases once immediate resuscitation has been initiated. Guidelines on neurosurgical referral are given in Section 5.4.

Aerocoele

Peri-orbital surgical emphysema (Section 2.5) suggests the presence of a fracture involving a skull sinus with associated intracranial air. This aerocele may expand if the nose is blown, thereby compressing adjacent brain tissue. Antibiotics should be started and the patient warned of the dangers associated with nose blowing. Early intracranial decompression is sometimes necessary, hence urgent discussion with a neurosurgeon is indicated.

Burr holes in the A and E department

Urgent decompression of the brain is essential when there is a rapidly developing acute extradural haematoma (Fig. 4.1). If a patient who was previously talking suddenly deteriorates there is an excellent potential for recovery because the primary brain injury is minimal [8]. To minimize further damage, specific treatment must be instituted urgently. This can be summarized as follows:

- Secure the airway, intubate and ventilate.
- Obtain i.v. access, check blood gases and cross-match blood.
- Contact a neurosurgeon – if it is decided to take the patient to theatre give i.v. Frusemide 80 mg or 20% Mannitol 1 g/kg infused over 10 to 15 minutes (i.e. 300–400 ml for an adult).
- Catheterize the bladder.
- If still awaiting transfer, shave the whole head.

If there is likely to be undue delay (greater than one hour) in reaching the neurosurgical unit and the deterioration continues despite the above measures then another surgeon may have to carry out burr holes in the Accident and Emergency

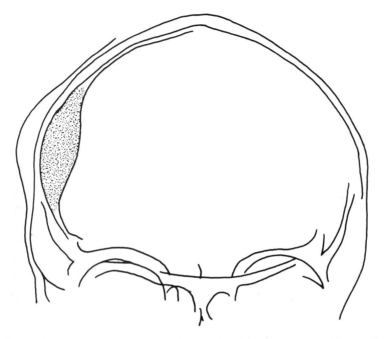

Fig. 4.1 Characteristic biconvex appearance of extradural haematoma with overlying scalp bruising.

department or in a nearby theatre. This is a temporizing measure which should ideally be carried out with the agreement of the neurosurgeon. It may be life-saving.

Burr holes: where to drill?

In the absence of a CT scan a clinical assessment of the site of the extradural haematoma must be made. The most likely area is underneath the scalp wound or close to the skull fracture. If there are localizing signs the haematoma is usually on the same side as the first dilating pupil (Section 2.8) and the opposite side to developing limb weakness. About three-quarters of extra-dural haematomas will be found in the temporo-parietal region. If in doubt the temporal site should be chosen for the first burr hole (Fig. 4.2).

Burr holes: how to do it?

Use the instruments shown in Fig. 4.3:

- Mark the elected site with a scratch before briefly cleaning and draping the scalp.

- Make a bold 2.5 cm long incision down to bone.

- Insert a self-retaining retractor. This will achieve haemostasis.

- Scrape aside the periosteum.

- Drill the hole by first using the perforator until the inner table is just breached. An extradural haematoma appears as dark red jelly-like blood between the inner table and the dura.

- Warn the anaesthetist that the

(continued)

(continued)

patient's level of consciousness may suddenly improve.

- Enlarge the hole with the burr and then if necessary by using bone nibblers.

- Control bleeding from the dural surface by surgicel and from the bone by bone wax.

- If no haematoma is obtained then further burr holes should be attempted. However, it is to be hoped that neurosurgical support will have arrived before this pepper-potting exercise is contemplated. More extensive exposure of a haematoma requires the expertise of a surgeon familiar with craniotomy.

- If there is a pale blue appearance of the dura this indicates the presence of a subdural haematoma. Seek neurosurgical advice before incising the dura.

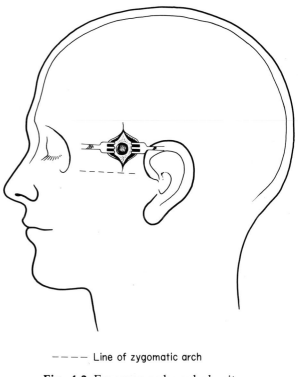

– – – – Line of zygomatic arch

Fig. 4.2 Emergency burr hole site.

4.3 SPECIFIC MANAGEMENT OF ACUTE PROBLEMS IN A AND E

Restlessness and aggression

Many head injured patients will present with a degree of disinhibition or bravado. This may be an expression of a personality trait but if it develops into more overt aggression it may be a reflection of a rising intracranial pressure or unassociated extracranial events. For example, the patient may have had a lot to drink before sustaining his head injury and now have a full bladder. Alcohol intoxication compounds this presentation. Hypoglycaemia may present in this way.

Assuming that the patient does not have a full bladder or diabetes, such behaviour should be tolerated and contained but not overtly suppressed. Any attempt to restrain the patient will usually cause more aggression.

Fits

The patient may be a known epileptic and have sustained the head injury during a normal fit. The after-effects of this seizure may still be present on admission. Occasionally a relatively minor head injury is associated with a grand mal fit but more

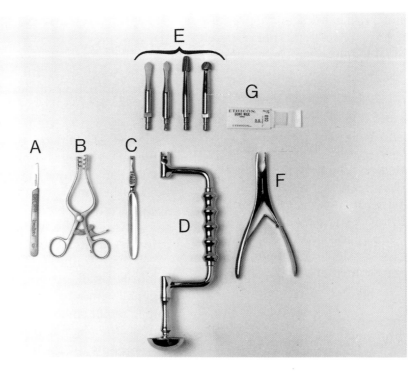

Fig. 4.3 Burr hole instruments; A scalpel; B West's self-retaining retractor; C periosteal elevator; D Hudson brace; E perforators and burrs; F bone nibblers; G bone wax.

commonly the latter is a complication of significant primary brain injury. In any event, continued epileptiform activity causes a significant rise in intracranial pressure and should be stopped immediately. Anoxia is a common and often unrecognized cause of epilepsy in such circumstances. The airway should be checked and 100% oxygen given. If the gag reflex is impaired endotracheal intubation is indicated. If the fitting is not judged to be due to anoxia, intravenous diazemuls (diazepam emulsion) should be given immediately. In small children when i.v. access proves difficult, the drug may be given rectally (as Stesolid 5–10 mg). Repeated seizures occurring despite the above measures may warrant the use of intravenous thiopentone (up to 500 mg), preferably administered by an anaesthetist. Prophylactic anticonvulsant drugs should also be given in this situation (Section 5.4).

Pain

The presence of a mild head injury must not preclude the adequate provision of analgesia to the patient with painful extracranial injuries. Neurological status is determined before giving small doses of intravenous opiates titrated against clinical response. Entonox (a mixture of 50% oxygen and 50% nitrous oxide) may be used initially when moving the injured patient and applying splints, but should not be given continuously. Nitrous oxide causes cerebral vasodilatation and a rise in intracranial pressure. The use of local anaesthetic nerve blocks can be invaluable in the management of rib and limb injuries.

Headache and anxiety

Simple oral analgesics (such as cocodaprin and paracetamol) which do not depress the conscious level can be given safely. This applies whether or not the patient is to be admitted. Intravenous diazemuls (diazepam emulsion) can occasionally be valuable to control the anxious uncooperative patient and allow further investigation and treatment.

Alcohol withdrawal

Head injured patients who present with acute alcohol intoxication or who have a history of alcohol abuse are at risk of developing withdrawal symptoms, commonly delirium tremens and seizures. Warning signs include tremor, anxiety, sweating and tachycardia. If this diagnosis is suspected, progression may be halted by the early administration of oral chlordiazepoxide (20–30 mg eight hourly) on a reducing dosage over a few days and a five-day course of intravenous vitamins B and C (Parentrovite).

Intraocular injury

Patients with blood in the anterior chamber (hyphaema) or evident retinal damage should be admitted for bed rest and the eye covered by a pad whilst awaiting an ophthalmic opinion.

4.4 MANAGEMENT OF SCALP WOUNDS

Having taken a careful history and made a brief examination of the scalp it should be possible to reconstruct the biomechanical forces applied to the head and to postulate the type of damage that will have been inflicted. This has implications for treatment. For example, a fall against a blunt hard surface may produce a stellate irregular scalp laceration which is usually amenable to cleansing in the A and E department and primary suture. Wounding by flying glass in a road traffic accident may result in multiple small lacerations, sometimes with a small amount of skin loss, and the impaction of small fragments of glass under the scalp. Again these can usually be managed in the A and E department, but sometimes an extensive search is required to remove all pieces of glass. These may have been driven under the scalp some distance from the wound.

A blow to the head for example by a weapon, a falling roof tile, or a golf club may cause a compound depressed vault fracture. As the patient often presents fully conscious and with no neurological signs, initial assessment may be misleading. In the case of assault the doctor's task may be hindered by the patient's reluctance to give an accurate history if he has been involved in criminal activities. Compound wounds will require in-patient care and should be examined cautiously in the A and E department.

Massive bleeding from the scalp is rare and usually stops spontaneously. In very small children it may be sufficient to warrant intravenous fluid therapy. The usual cause of prolonged bleeding in an adult is anti-coagulant therapy or continued washing and meddling with the wound by concerned relatives or friends. On arrival, patients with large or briskly bleeding wounds should be placed on a tipping trolley beside a good light. Sterile gloved hands are required to assess the scalp and to stop bleeding by digital pressure (see Fig. 4.6). Hair in the immediate vicinity of the wound is cut away after discussion with the patient. The area is then cleaned with aqueous chlorhexidine solution. If necessary a light dressing is applied or a few approximating haemostatic sutures inserted before the patient is sent for skull X-ray. Remember that the wound, matted hair and the dressing may mimic a fracture on the radiograph.

Definitive treatment should start with shaving of the scalp for at least 2 cm on either side of the wound. Re-examination at this time will usually enable a more precise assessment of the wounding mechanism to be made, this in turn determining the direction of search required for embedded foreign bodies and dirt.

Anaesthesia

Local infiltration with 1% plain Lignocaine is usually adequate for modest scalp wounds. Lignocaine 1% with adrenaline may be used for extensive wounds as larger volumes can be safely given and coincidentally it reduces bleeding. The toxic effects of Lignocaine include convulsions, bradycardia and cardiac arrest so it is important to be aware of the recommended safe adult dose – less than 20 ml of 1% plain Lignocaine and less than 50 ml of 1% Lignocaine plus adrenaline. Remember to check by aspiration that the needle is not in a vessel.

The solution is most conveniently injected subcutaneously through the wound edge. Alternatively nerve blocks can be used. This technique is quicker, less painful and avoids further distortion and swelling of the wound when a small volume is injected around a subcutaneous nerve (Figs. 4.4 and 4.5). Supra-trochlea and supra-orbital blocks can be combined to anaesthetize the commonly injured frontal region for a distance of at least 10 cm above the eyebrow. These nerves can be blocked bilaterally if necessary from a single injection site in the nasal bridge. The needle is directed downwards and laterally towards the medial canthus and then directed laterally under the supra-orbital rim. About 1–2 ml is adequate and should be deposited on either side of the supra-orbital notch.

For very extensive wounds it may be possible to completely anaesthetize the scalp by circumferential nerve blocks. However when this is not possible, for example in a young child, a general anaesthetic is more appropriate. The latter may have to be delayed because of recent food and drink intake. In this case a temporary occlusive dressing should be applied after wound cleansing, and systemic antibiotics considered.

Exploration and wound toilet

Bleeding will have recommenced during this exploratory and cleaning process but will usually be arrested by scalp sutures. If bleeding is severe it can be stopped temporarily by digital compression of the scalp (Fig. 4.6) or by use of a West's self-retaining retractor (Fig. 4.7). Use of a bipolar diathermy is helpful as it causes minimal

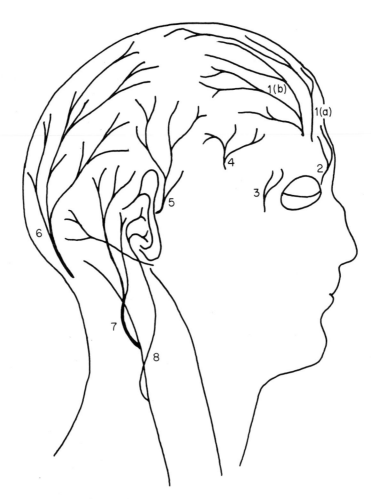

Fig. 4.4 Cutaneous nerves supplying the scalp – lateral view. 1. supraorbital nerve, a) = medial branch, b) = lateral branch, 2 = supratrochlear nerve, 3 = zygomaticofacial nerve, 4 = zygomaticotemporal nerve, 5 = auriculotemporal nerve, 6 = greater occipital nerve, 7 = lesser occipital nerve, 8 = greater auricular nerve.

damage to surrounding tissue whilst co-agulating the vessel between the forceps. Wounds more than 2 cm long should be explored gently using a sterile gloved finger, noting the state of the skin edge, aponeurosis and skull. Findings should be recorded as in Fig. 4.8.

It is unusual for the scalp to be completely devascularized during injury and therefore excision of apparently contused and necrotic skin should not be undertaken lightly. If an unsuspected vault fracture is detected at this stage further exploration should be deferred until a neurosurgical opinion has been sought. Closure is achieved in layers once the wound has been thoroughly cleaned and all foreign bodies and dirt removed, if necessary by painstaking

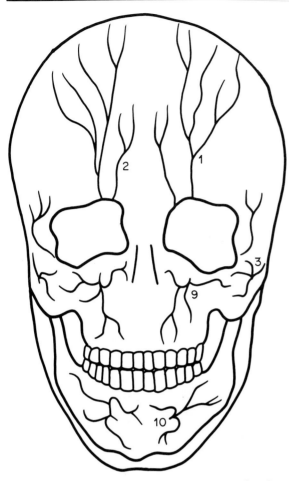

Fig. 4.5 Cutaneous nerves supplying the face and scalp – anterior view. 1 = supraorbital nerve, 2 = supratrochlear nerve, 3 = zygomaticofacial nerve, 9 = infraorbital nerve, 10 = mental nerve.

sharp dissection with scalpel and toothed forceps.

Closure

An attempt should be made to close the galea with an absorbable suture (e.g. chromic catgut) followed by interrupted silk sutures into the scalp skin. If this is not possible vertical mattress sutures should be used in an attempt to close the 'dead space' (Fig. 4.9).

For the hairy scalp 3/0 silk should be used routinely but 2/0 silk on a hand needle may be preferable for deep mattress sutures; 5/0 or 6/0 monofilament nylon is preferable for the forehead and face. Adhesive strips can be used for small superficial wounds especially on the forehead of children. Some superficial scalp lacerations can be adequately closed by judicious tying of adjacent strands of hair.

Never shave the eyebrows, even if there are underlying lacerations. They offer good anatomical guidelines for cosmetic reconstruction. Wounds of the eyelids demand exact reconstitution, particularly if they involve the lid margins. Injuries to the lid margins should always be referred to a plastic surgeon or ophthalmologist.

The head should be washed before the patient leaves the A and E department. The patient will be advised not to wash his hair or get the wound wet until after the time for suture removal (about seven days). Although general dirt associated with an accident can be washed away during the initial stages of wound inspection, subsequent bleeding into the hair during wound closure demands that a second scalp wash be carried out after wound closure with an antiseptic solution, e.g. Betadine (Povidine iodine). Small wounds can then usually be left without a dressing although some advocate the use of a plastic spray or other sealant. More extensive wounds will benefit from a pressure dressing to prevent haematoma formation.

Anti-tetanus prophylaxis should be given where appropriate and antibiotics prescribed for compound or basal skull fractures.

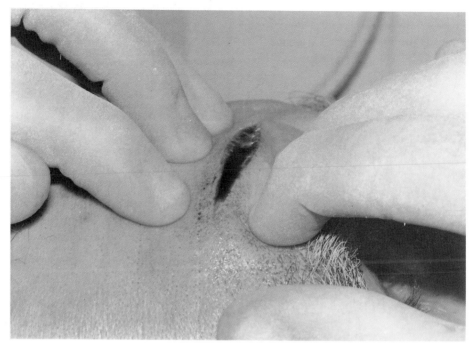

Fig. 4.6 Digital control of scalp bleeding.

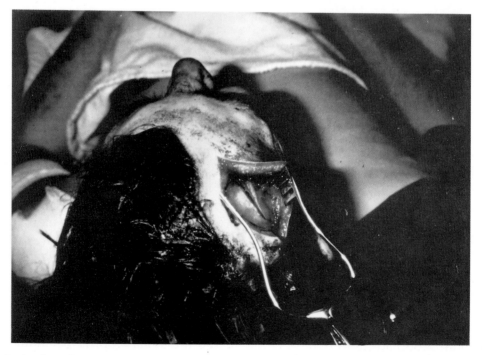

Fig. 4.7 Incised scalp wound showing use of West's self-retaining retractor for exploration and haemostasis.

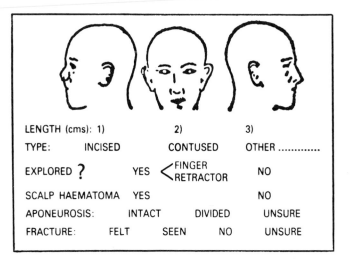

LENGTH (cms): 1)   2)   3)

TYPE: INCISED   CONTUSED   OTHER ....

EXPLORED **?**   YES <FINGER   NO
                          RETRACTOR

SCALP HAEMATOMA   YES   NO

APONEUROSIS: INTACT   DIVIDED   UNSURE

FRACTURE: FELT   SEEN   NO   UNSURE

Fig. 4.8 Scalp stamp.

4.5 TO ADMIT OR NOT TO ADMIT?

The A and E doctor's main concern is to decide whether or not the patient should be admitted for a period of observation. Patients who are confused or have other evident impairment to the level of consciousness, exhibit neurological deterioration or have focal neurological signs are likely to have sustained primary brain injury and will require at least a period of hospital observation. However, patients who have none of the above features may go on to develop 'secondary brain injury' for the reasons listed in Table 4.1. The cardiorespiratory aspects of secondary deterioration have been discussed in Sections 4.1 and 4.2. Here we are more concerned with the early detection and prevention of deterioration due to intracranial haematoma (Section 4.2), brain swelling and infection.

Up to 3% of all patients attending A and E with a head injury will have a skull fracture, and about one out of every 30 adults with a recent skull fracture will have an acute extradural haematoma. If the conscious level is reduced the risk is 1 in 4 [5].

Skull fracture can only occur with direct 'impact' damage to the head. The energy required to fracture the skull at impact may go on to inflict considerable primary brain damage or lead to secondary brain damage because the bone fracture may lacerate local meningeal blood vessels leading to extradural haemorrhage. In contrast, deceleration/acceleration or 'impulsive' forces may inflict considerable primary brain damage (diffuse axonal injury) without major damage to the skull or scalp, i.e. without skull fracture.

The detection of skull fracture is therefore an important indication of the risk of extradural haematoma development. Patients with clinical signs of basal skull fracture (such as bleeding from the ears or nose or peri-orbital haematoma) must be admitted.

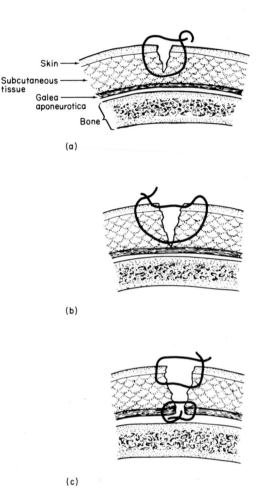

Fig. 4.9 Closure of scalp lacerations: (a) superficial wound. Minimal bleeding; (b) deep wound, aponeurosis intact; (c) deep wound with divided aponeurosis.

along with those who are found to have vault fractures on skull radiography. If radiography cannot be obtained for technical or staffing reasons, yet the patient has fulfilled the requirements for skull radiography, a period of in-patient observation is essential. It is unwise to ask a patient to 'come back in the morning for an X-ray', by which time the most critical period for potential deterioration will have passed. Similarly, it is essential to err on the side of caution when interpreting poor quality films (or if you are a poor quality interpreter!). If in doubt admit.

However, it would be unwise to admit every head injured patient who comes to the A and E department. Although neurological observation for a period of 24 hours in all such cases might appear to be a counsel of perfection, this policy would result in the great majority of admitted patients making an uneventful recovery. Not only is this expensive in terms of hospital resources and extremely disruptive for the majority of patients, it is also counterproductive. There would be an increased threshold for the recognition of neurological abnormality if medical and nursing staff routinely saw large numbers of patients making uneventful recoveries.

Indications for admission

Table 4.2 lists the indications for admission of the apparently uncomplicated mild head injury. This is based upon the authors' experience and guidelines proposed by a 'Group of Neurosurgeons' [9] When there is some uncertainty, particularly about domestic support, the conditions pertaining at home must be compared with the facilities available in the hospital for continuing careful neurological observation. This dilemma is considered in more detail in Section 5.6.

Most important observations relate to changes in behaviour and in level of consciousness (Section 4.2). Occasionally, focal signs may be elicited which appear to be inappropriate to the level of consciousness.

Table 4.2 Admission/discharge policy

Admit if ANY of the following obtain
1. Post-traumatic amnesia more than 5 min or no recall of the incident
2. Reduced conscious level or abnormal behaviour
3. Clinical or radiological evidence of vault fracture
4. Clinical evidence of basal fracture
5. Focal neurological signs
6. Severe or increasing headache
7. Vomiting within 12 hours of examination
8. Special risk (anticoagulants, haemophilia, hydrocephalus)
9. Difficulty in assessment (e.g. in epileptic, drunk or child)
10. Persisting nausea, dizziness or other symptoms
11. Inadequate history
12. Inadequate domestic support

They may be longstanding, particularly in elderly patients. For example there may be irregular pupils due to previous cataract surgery or limb weakness and incoordination due to an earlier head injury or cerebrovascular accident. Providing the patient or relative can give a good account of this previous disability and no recent change is apparent, it should be noted and then disregarded as a factor for admission.

Other more acute neurological signs may be detected in the fully conscious patient which are not related to brain injury. For example a lower motor neurone type facial palsy may be the immediate or delayed result of a fracture of the petrous temporal bone. This may be associated with ipsilateral deafness, haemotympanum and leakage of CSF or blood from the ear. These patients should be referred for neurosurgical or ENT advice (repair of the facial nerve within the bony canal may occasionally be appropriate). Numbness or altered sensation in the face may be associated with facial injury (Section 2.5).

Limb weakness or sensory disturbance may be caused by spinal as well as cerebral injury. Appropriate X-rays should be carried out and the spine stabilized before considering transfer to a neurosurgical unit.

Mild headache, transient nausea and dizziness are commonplace after minor head injury. Their presence must prompt a very thorough examination to exclude positive clinical signs. If the patient is found to be fit in all other respects (Table 4.2) the presence of these mild symptoms need not preclude discharge.

Headache which is severe or increasing and unrelieved by simple analgesics may indicate raised intracranial pressure and therefore justifies admission in its own right.

Vomiting alone is rarely an early sign of raised intracranial pressure. More often it is an indication of a damaged vestibular mechanism (with or without a petrous temporal fracture) or simply a measure of a degree of brain 'shake-up'. The threshold for vomiting is low in children and those under the influence of alcohol. Admission is advised for all with persisting nausea, or who have vomited within twelve hours of examination. Admission allows rest and appropriate treatment of associated gastritis or peptic ulceration as well as neurological observation.

Dizziness by itself is not an absolute indication for admission. Mild intermittent vertigo induced by sudden changes of head and neck position may be managed on an out-patient basis. Those with severe vertigo may require complete bed rest in hospital. Elderly patients who were prone to dizzy spells prior to the head injury may warrant in-patient investigation to establish the cause. Further falls may be preventable.

Other symptoms, often persisting and distressing, e.g. visual disturbances or slurred speech, often resolve within a few hours. However a period of observation can be reassuring to both doctor and patient and the rest should speed resolution of symptoms.

Amnesia

There is still some debate concerning what length of post-traumatic amnesia (PTA) or history of unconsciousness (if any) is associated with an increased risk of intracranial haematoma. The authors believe that PTA, in particular, is useful as a guide to the severity of the head injury and recommend admission if:

(a) The patient cannot recall the circumstances

The circumstances of the injury cannot be recalled due to retrograde amnesia. For example, a patient may recall going out drinking and later discover that he has sustained a scalp wound. His amnesia for the incident may be entirely or at least in part due to effects of alcohol. Nevertheless, the casualty officer should assume that this head injury is the prime cause of the amnesia and should recommend a period of observation.

(b) Post-traumatic amnesia is greater than five minutes

If there are no reliable witnesses to the timing of the injury and the patient's subsequent behaviour, the length of PTA may be difficult to determine. Consider a man who leaves a public house at 11 pm. He recalls stepping off the pavement, seeing the headlights of a car approaching, feeling the thud of the impact, waking up at the side of the road and being taken to hospital. His post-traumatic amnesia could have been a few seconds or as long as a few hours depending upon how long it took for help to arrive.

Assessment of amnesia may be impossible not only in the alcohol abuser but also in the epileptic, the elderly demented patient or the young child.

Inability to determine the length of amnesia casts doubt upon the severity of injury and it is wise to admit such patients unless there is reliable evidence that the injury was trivial.

Special risks

Risks such as those associated with haemophilia or, more commonly, anticoagulant therapy, should always be considered. Such patients must be admitted even following very minor blows to the head. The appropriate physician should be contacted regarding medication. Hydrocephalic patients are also at special risk. Their management should be discussed with a neurosurgeon.

Children

Parents are often concerned at the tendency of their child to go to sleep after a minor head injury. This may occur during the day but is commoner in the evening, often reflecting the fact that the child has been kept awake in the A and E department after normal bedtime. The parents should be advised not to be alarmed by this and not to try to keep their child awake. They should, however, ensure that there is a normal response to a mild verbal or tactile stimulation. This will vary from child to child and any subtle alteration in sleep pattern will be more readily detected by caring parents than by hospital doctors or nurses.

If during this conversation with the parents or patient and third party, there is any expression of anxiety about home management, it is advisable to admit the patient.

4.6 ADVICE TO RELATIVES AND FRIENDS

Those accompanying the patient should be kept informed about progress at all stages. Clearly this is particularly important when the patient may be discharged into their care. Never discuss out-patient management with the patient alone. It is essential that a third party is aware of the potential complications and will accompany the patient home. An instruction card similar to

---

St. Elsewhere's Hospital

Accident and Emergency department
Tel: 001 775 533, ext 2173

Head Injury Warning

Name: ....
Address: ....
received treatment for a head injury on ....

    If you notice any of the following changes in the patient's condition telephone the hospital **AT ONCE** and ask to speak to the Casualty Officer or bring the patient to the Accident and Emergency Department.
1. Increasing drowsiness or confusion
2. Severe headache
3. Weakness of an arm or leg
4. Vomiting
5. Leakage from the ear or nose

Fig. 4.10 Head injury advice form.

that shown in Fig. 4.10 should be given to the patient or parent and its safe receipt recorded by a signature in the clinical notes (see also Section 5.6).

It is also helpful to advise relatives and friends about the reasons for a short period of in-patient observation and the modifications of behaviour that can be expected for the first few days after discharge from hospital with a minor head injury. They should be advised that the patient may be tired and irritable and may feel inadequate when trying to get back to his or her previous activities of daily living. These aspects of care are discussed in detail in Chapter 6.

Box 4

CASE HISTORY

A 25-year old man is brought to the A and E department by ambulance having sustained apparently mild head injuries after his car went out of control. On examination he is somewhat disinhibited but has no focal neurological signs and is considered to have 'three top lines' on the Glasgow Coma Scale. There is a minor right parietal scalp contusion and a seat belt mark over the upper right anterior chest wall.

Fifteen minutes after arrival his level of consciousness deteriorates rapidly. He responds only to painful stimuli, displays marked left-sided weakness and has a dilated unresponsive left pupil.

What is your differential diagnosis and immediate management?

Intracranial haematoma/hypotension and hypoxia/hypoglycaemia/epileptic fit?

Rapid re-examination reveals normal blood pressure, good perfusion and no evidence of systemic injury. Subsequent chest and skull radiographs are normal. Injection marks are found on the thighs. Blood sugar is 1.5 mmol/l (normal range 3.0 to 6.0 mmol/l). Intravenous injection of 100 ml of 50% glucose immediately reverses all neurological signs. CT scan is normal.

This man probably became drowsy at the wheel due to mild hypoglycaemia. Subsequently he lost control of his car. No other vehicle was involved in the accident. The hyperglycaemic response to injury would cause a temporary reversal of the hypoglycaemia, hence the disinhibited behaviour on arrival. As this glucose was metabolized, clinical signs of hypoglycaemia reappeared. These are not always global and can mimic focal neurological deterioration in the manner described above.

Golden rule

Always consider diabetes as a cause of deterioration in head injured patients.

4.7 REFUSAL OF TREATMENT

It is not uncommon for patients to refuse treatment. These people are usually victims of assault and under the influence of alcohol or drugs. They may appear to be uncooperative (and ungrateful!) and give no good reason for their action. However, the underlying problem is likely to be fear of needles, hospitals, police, further assault or alcohol/drug withdrawal.

How hard should one try to persuade a patient to comply with treatment? If the condition is potentially life-threatening, e.g. severe scalp bleeding, then reasonable restraint (if necessary with the help of the police) may be justified in order to insert a few deep haemostatic sutures. Refusal of wound exploration or skull X-ray means that a compound fracture may be missed. In this case antibiotic therapy and admission should be offered as a reasonable compromise.

'Refusal of treatment' forms may be signed by the patient but they should not be used as an alternative to listening sympathetically to the patient's point of view in private.

Whenever treatment is refused and particularly if it is enforced against the patient's will attempts should be made to inform a relative. The details should be recorded and witnessed by two senior members of the Accident and Emergency staff.

5 In-patient management

The decision to admit a patient with a minor head injury must take into account not only the clinical features discussed in earlier chapters, but also the comparative benefits of observation at home and in hospital. The prerequisites for home surveillance are discussed in Section 5.6. It is equally important to appreciate the level of care which can be offered to those who are admitted for hospital observation. The provision of facilities – and, more importantly, nursing staff and doctors – may be inadequate in some parts of the hospital.

It is essential that admitting wards are appropriately staffed by nurses trained in neurological observation and the use of the Glasgow Coma Scale. Medical staff must review and 'clerk in' the patient, once on the ward and not merely accept the A and E department record. A plan of care must be agreed between medical and nursing staff and discussed with the patient and relatives or friends.

Many hospitals in the UK now have 'short stay' or 'observation' wards. Beds therein are commonly used and controlled by A and E staff. Whatever the local arrangement, it is essential that there is a continuum of care between the A and E department, the ward and the local neurosurgical service. This should be planned and developed in the cold light of day and not debated in the small hours when trying to defend the delayed transfer of a patient with an expanding extradural haemorrhage.

5.1 CHILDREN

Examination of young children, in particular those less than five years of age, can be difficult in the environment of the A and E department. A separate area for examination of children may help to reduce distress. The child should be sensitively but thoroughly examined for extracranial injuries, paying particular attention to skin marks, bruising, the eyes, ears and mouth.

If injuries are discovered which are not consistent with the story given and there is a possibility of child abuse, senior advice should be sought. The parents or guardians should be informed that admission is necessary on clinical grounds and for further investigation of the nature of the injuries. Photographs and skeletal surveys should not be arranged in the A and E department and the possibility of abuse should not be discussed. This is best left for the paediatrician and social worker, once the child is on the paediatric ward.

The **Glasgow Coma Scale** is primarily

intended for assessement of adults. In children an accurate interpretation of the verbal response may be impossible to obtain and a modified version of the **Glasgow Coma Scale** may be helpful (Table 5.1; Section 5.3). A most valuable aid in assessment is of course the opinion of the mother or other close relative who should recognize abnormal behaviour in her children better than the doctor or nurse. Persisting concern by a mother should be a major factor influencing admission and must never be ignored. Apart from the likelihood that she may be right about her child's condition, reassurance of a distraught parent can be very difficult and time-consuming. Admission on 'social grounds' is often worthwhile in these cases.

Conversely, children under 16 years of age who present with minor head injuries should not be allowed home without the knowledge and consent of their parents, even if they fulfil all the other criteria for discharge listed in Table 4.2 (Section 4.5). It is wise to admit them to a short stay observation area or paediatric ward pending the arrival of a responsible adult.

Whenever admission is indicated there should be facilities for the child's mother to stay overnight. Parents or guardians should not be told that their child 'will definitely be allowed home in the morning' even if this is very likely. They should be made aware, however, that this is possible depending upon further assessment.

5.2 THE ELDERLY

Many elderly people live alone and the circumstance of their accident may not have

Table 5.1 A suggested Paediatric Coma Scale

Eyes open	
Spontaneously	4
To speech	3
To pain	2
None	1
Best verbal response*	
Normal words or sounds	5
Abnormal words or sounds	3
None	1
Best motor response	
Obeys or plays†	6
Localizes pain	5
Flexion to pain	3
Extension to pain	2
None	1

* For children too young to allow assessment of orientation
† 'Play' is used in the broadest sense e.g. 'shaking a rattle' or 'refusing to give back the doctor's pen torch'. Neonates and some young infants may have a 'top line' of less than 6 according to their stage of development.

been witnessed. Admission is always indicated in these cases on the assumption that the history is unreliable and the domestic support for follow-up at home is inadequate. Subsequent discharge to caring relatives may be possible once the cause and nature of the injuries have been investigated. Whenever there is a suggestion of a fall or dizziness, a full assessment is indicated. Possible causes include cardiovascular disease, respiratory tract infection, diabetes, thyroid disease, neurological problems, cervical spondylosis, alcohol abuse and inappropriate medication (Table 1.1; Section 1.4). A pelvic radiograph and anteroposterior and lateral X-rays of the hip should be taken to exclude fracture of the femoral neck.

The blood pressure will have been measured in the routine assessment of the patient's head injury. In the elderly patient it is important to check the fundi for hypertensive retinopathy also. If admission is indicated, based on the more sensitive criteria outlined above, the following investigations must be carried out as a matter of routine: chest X-ray, ECG, full blood count, urea and electrolytes, blood sugar and urinalysis. Thyroid function tests may be indicated. If there is any suggestion of the recent onset of confusion (within the past few months) a chronic subdural haematoma should be excluded by a period of observation and/or brain scan (see Section 5.3).

Social problems in the elderly

Some patients present with trivial head injuries but major social problems. Admission for assessment is advisable if there is no domestic support and the general practitioner and social services cannot offer immediate assistance. Physiotherapy and appropriate nursing care during such an admission will often improve the patient's ability to cope subsequently at home. If this is unsuccessful, early involvement of occupational therapist, social worker, geriatric specialist and general practitioner is essential so that long-term care can be planned. Ideally this group should be informed when the patient is in the A and E department as it might be possible to avoid acute admission altogether by arranging more appropriate community care.

5.3 OBSERVATION

Patients with apparently mild head injuries should be admitted to wards situated close to the A and E department particularly if medical staff from that department are involved in their supervision. It is most important that experienced nursing and medical staff are available in adequate numbers throughout the night and day. Admitting doctors should speak to the nurse-in-charge, giving details both of the reason for admission and the required management. Ideally both nurse and doctor should examine the patient shortly after his or her arrival on the ward and should together check the conscious level and relevant neurological signs. With change over of medical and nursing staff, it is important to maintain continuity of patient assessment. Nursing staff have a formal 'change-over report' and it is good practice for the doctor coming on duty to be similarly up-dated on the progress of the patients by way of a brief ward round conducted by the retiring doctor.

Documentation

This may be regarded as a chore by some but it is an essential part of management. Misunder-standing can be avoided by writing brief notes summarizing the diagnosis and agreed plan of management. Examples are given in Fig. 5.1.

An observation chart (Fig 5.2) used by nursing staff who clearly understand the Glasgow Coma Scale and other neurological observations is the cornerstone of early detection of neurological deterioration.

Observation is commenced and findings recorded on the chart when the patient is

---

1. Diagnosis: Assault, right parietal scalp laceration,
                  disorientated, no skull fracture.

    Requires: Suture scalp
                 Half-hourly neurological observations.

2. Diagnosis: Epileptic seizure × 1 at 8pm, still 'post-ictal' at
                 8.30pm.
                 Known alcoholic.
                 Abrasion of occiput but no skull fracture evident.
                 i.v. cannula in situ.

    Requires: Constant observation, oxygen therapy (100%)
                 Contact neurosurgeons – transfer if either
                        further fit
                        or incomplete recovery from this fit.
                 I will review in half an hour.

Fig. 5.1 Examples of documentation.

first examined in the A and E department. The chart (or a photocopy) stays with the patient during admission to the observation ward or transfer to a neurosurgical unit. The three responses of the Coma Scale (Section 2.6) should be recorded with interconnected dots (as in a temperature chart) to show the pattern of progress at a glance (Fig. 5.2). Ticks should not be used. An alternative chart for children includes the modified version of the Glasgow Coma Scale (Table 5.1; Section 5.1).

The conscious level normally varies throughout a 24-hour period. This should be recorded on the observation chart. The repeated recording of 'eyes open spontaneously' (Fig. 5.3) throughout the night and day usually indicates that the nurse does not understand the correct method of assessment, i.e. observation begins by looking at and not by speaking to or touching the patient.

Only by a meticulous approach can subtle features such as 'altered sleep pattern' be seen, a finding which may be an early indication of raised intracranial pressure. (Fig. 5.4).

Frequency and duration of observation

A plan relating frequency and duration of observation to presenting signs and symptoms is described in Table 5.2. The risk of a rapid deterioration due to an intracranial haematoma is greatest during the first 24 hours after injury. Certain features increase the likelihood of this complication, e.g. patients with a skull fracture and disorientation have a one in four risk. Fig. 5.5 lists those features which demand consultation with a neurosurgeon and indicate their relative urgency. This is discussed more fully in Section 5.4.

GLASGOW ROYAL INFIRMARY

OBSERVATION CHART

NAME

RECORD No.

DATE: ←13/11/87→ - - - - - - - 17/11/87 - - 23/11/87

TIME: 17 20 | 17 40 | 18 20 | 18 45 | 19 10 | 19 15 | 19 20 | 19 40

COMA SCALE			
Eyes open	Spontaneously		Eyes closed by swelling = C
	To speech		
	To pain		
	None		
Best verbal response	Orientated		Endotracheal tube or tracheostomy = T
	Confused		
	Inappropriate Words		
	Incomprehensible Sounds		
	None		
Best motor response	Obey commands		Usually record the best arm response
	Localise pain		
	Flexion to pain		
	Extension to pain		
	None		

A   B   C

Pupil scale (m.m.): 1, 2, 3, 4, 5, 6, 7, 8

Blood pressure and Pulse rate: 240 230 220 210 200 190 180 170 160 150 140 130 120 110 100 90 80 70 60 50 40 30 20 10

Temperature °C: 40 39 38 37 36 35 34 33 32 31 30

Respiration

ARRIVAL   TRANSFER   CRANIOTOMY   DISCHARGE

PUPILS															
right	Size	3	3	4	3	4	4		8	-	-	-	4	-	4
	Reaction	+	+	+	+	+	+		-				+		+
left	Size	3	3	4	3	4		8	-	-	-		4	-	4
	Reaction	+	+	+	+	+		-					+		+

+ reacts
− no reaction
c. eye closed

LIMB MOVEMENT			
ARMS	Normal power		Record right (R) and left (L) separately if there is a difference between the two sides
	Mild weakness		
	Severe weakness		
	Spastic flexion		
	Extension		
	No response		
LEGS	Normal power		
	Mild weakness		
	Severe weakness		
	Extension		
	No response		

ARRIVAL   TRANSFER   CRANIOTOMY   DISCHARGE

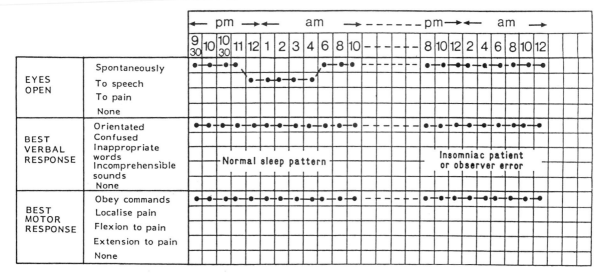

Fig. 5.3 Sleep patterns.

Patients awaiting transfer must be kept under constant observation. The remaining patients should be observed at half-hourly intervals for the first two hours after arrival in the A and E Department. This allows the ward nursing staff to become quickly familiar with the patient and his or her neurological status. If there is a skull fracture or there is repeated vomiting, severe headache, focal neurological signs or depressed consciousness, i.e. the patient is considered to be in the 'moderate risk group', then half-hourly observations should be continued. If any of these features persist eight

Fig. 5.2 (opposite page) Example of early development of extradural haematoma.

A 12 year old boy fell from the back of a moving bus. He was taken quickly by ambulance to hospital. On arrival at A and E, he was orientated but did not recall the accident. He had left frontotemporal scalp bruising and was bleeding from his left ear.

X-rays of the chest, neck and skull were normal but i.v. penicillin and sulphadimidine were given on the assumption that he had a basal skull fracture.

One hour after arrival he became confused but he had no localizing neurological signs. A neurosurgeon was contacted, transfer was agreed and arterial blood gas analysis carried out. However, before transfer could be effected, further rapid deterioration occurred. He was intubated and ventilated and an i.v. Mannitol infusion commenced.

Despite these measures, by the time craniotomy was performed there was no motor response and both pupils were fixed and dilated. A large left-sided extradural haematoma was evacuated. Fortunately he made an excellent recovery and was fit for discharge after ten days. When reviewed one month after the accident his left hemiparesis had resolved and he had normal speech and hearing. His mild behaviour problems and difficulty in concentrating were improving and he was keen to return to school. He was subsequently able to resume normal school work without difficulty.

		← pm →	← am →	← pm →	← am →
		7:30 8 8:30 9 10 11 12 1	2 4 6 8 10 12 2 4	6 8 10 12 2 4 6 8	10 12 2 4 6 8 10 12 1
EYES OPEN	Spontaneously				T
	To speech				R
	To pain				A
	None				N
BEST VERBAL RESPONSE	Normal words or sounds				S
	Abnormal words or sounds				F
	None				E
BEST MOTOR RESPONSE	Obey commands				R
	Localise pain				R
	Flexion to pain				E
	Extension to pain				D
	None				

Fig. 5.4 Example of delayed detection of extradural haematoma.

A three year old boy was knocked down by a car at low speed. He suffered bruising of his arms and legs but his main injury was a temporal skull fracture. He vomited several times after arrival at the A and E department and was crying. He was admitted to the paediatric ward and although his level of consciousness quickly returned to normal he did not sleep well. On the folllowing day he was 'tired' and was nursed in bed.

On the next day he was able to walk around and he ate his breakfast. His mother was keen to take him home but at midday the nursing staff found that he was acting and talking strangely. His mother agreed that he was unusually quiet and 'not his usual self'. Although the doctor found no other abnormal neurological signs transfer to the neurosurgical unit was arranged and a large extradural haematoma was evacuated.

hours after arrival then neurosurgical advice should be sought. Otherwise the frequency of observation can gradually be reduced (Table 5.2).

Most patients should be observed for a minimum of 12 hours and should be thoroughly examined thereafter (Fig. 5.6). This provides an opportunity to check the patient's recollection of events before and after the incident, to check the nature and severity of the injury and to establish whether a full recovery has been made. Patients who have vomited within the 12 hours before this examination should be advised to remain at least until they have managed to 'keep down some hospital food' (a good test of the constitution). Headache which is satisfactorily relieved by two Cocodaprin tablets is not an indication for further observation. More severe headache should be taken seriously and may warrant referral to a neurosurgeon.

Patients with a skull fracture should be detained for a minimum of 48 hours after the time of injury. Those with a basal skull fracture who for some reason are not transferred to a neurosurgical ward, require bed rest and observation until there has

Table 5.2

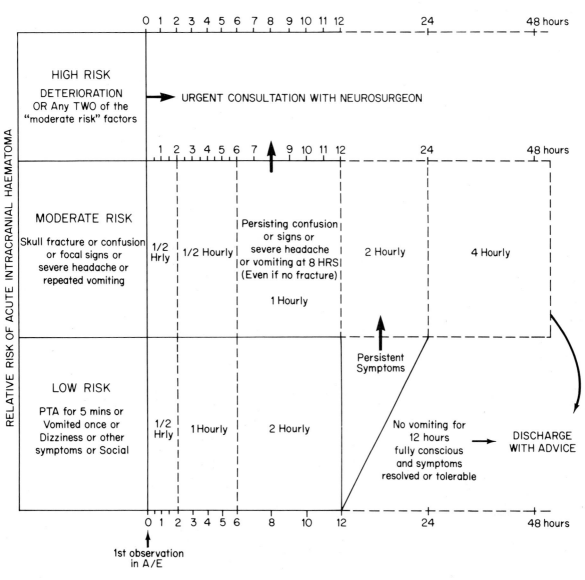

been no CSF leak for 48 hours, and symptoms, e.g. vertigo, have become manageable. This usually requires at least five days' admission. Antibiotic therapy should be continued for five days after the CSF leak has stopped and discharge should not be considered unless home circumstances allow complete rest in bed for at least one week.

The 'special risk' patient (Section 4.5) with bleeding diathesis or hydrocephalus should be regarded as at least in the

Immediate
1. Coma continuing after resuscitation
2. Deterioration of conscious level
                or of neurological signs
3. Epileptic fit with skull fracture
                or without complete recovery
4. Any combination of the following:

Skull fracture	Depressed conscious level
Severe headache or repeated vomiting	Acute focal neurological signs

Soon
5. Confusion or other neurological disturbance persisting after 8 hours
6. Compound depressed fracture of the vault
7. Suspected basal skull fracture

Fig. 5.5 Criteria for consultation with a neurosurgeon.

Date: / /	Time:			
PTA (min)	No	<5;	5–60;	>60
Vomited in past 12 h	No	Yes		
Headache present	No	Mild	Severe	
Other symptoms	No	Yes _____		
Neurological signs	No	Yes _____		
Glasgow Coma Scale	E	M	V	

Fig. 5.6 Ward stamp.

moderate risk category and observed as indicated above. The threshold for neurosurgical referral in such cases should be lowered.

A patient who has a history of symptoms which have slowly developed several days or weeks after a head injury may be suffering from a chronic subdural haematoma (Section 5.2). If there is disorientation or focal signs, admission will be necessary for urgent investigation, e.g isotope brain scan or CT scan. In other cases a period of observation may be of value in establishing the sleep pattern and the presence of abnormal fluctuations in consciousness. In such cases initial observation at a frequency of every two to four hours will be sufficient to establish objective evidence to present to a neurosurgeon.

Rest and posture

Patients with basal skull fracture, intraocular injury or facial swelling are best managed sitting up in bed. This should help to reduce swelling, control intracranial pressure and minimize further intraocular damage or CSF leak. Those with headache should not be denied simple analgesia (Section 4.3) and should rest in the quietest area of the ward.

Management of the intoxicated patient with bleeding scalp wounds presents considerable problems to the nursing staff. When he awakes to find himself in a hospital ward he has a full bladder and may be hypovolaemic, hypoglycaemic and anaemic. If he attempts to walk unaided to the toilet or shower, he is likely to have a syncopal attack (and suffer another injury). He should be encouraged to sit up slowly and use a urine bottle. A cup of tea may restore his vitality – but remember to have a vomit bowl handy!

5.4 CONSULTATION WITH A NEUROSURGEON

Criteria for neurosurgical consultation should be worked out and agreed between every A and E department and its neurosurgical referral centre. This applies as much when the two departments are in the same building as when they are many miles apart. The threshold for consultation will inevitably vary according to the expertise and facilities in the primary hospital and the time taken to transfer to the neurosurgical centre. Remote hospitals may have surgeons who are prepared to evacuate extradural haematomas. Sometimes this is necessary. This is becoming a less frequent event however with the introduction of the CT scanner, the more liberal policy for transfer of patients before deterioration has commenced, and the availability of the helicopter.

The four **high risk** patient groups requiring urgent consultation are outlined in Fig. 5.5.

Coma

The patient who is in 'coma' (E1, M5, V2 or worse) on arrival and subsequently remains so despite restoration of his cardiorespiratory state, may benefit from neurosurgical care. It is however most important that other serious conditions which may contribute to the clinical picture, e.g. hypoglycaemia, haemopneumothorax, ruptured spleen or spinal injury, are excluded or dealt with before transfer. Sometimes a multiply injured patient is not fit for transfer and a neurosurgeon may be required to come to the primary hospital in order to assess and operate on the patient. In severe alcohol intoxication, where there are no localizing signs, no skull fracture and minimal injury to the scalp, the most appropriate neurosurgical advice may be to continue supportive therapy and careful observation (Fig. 5.7). Conscious level and

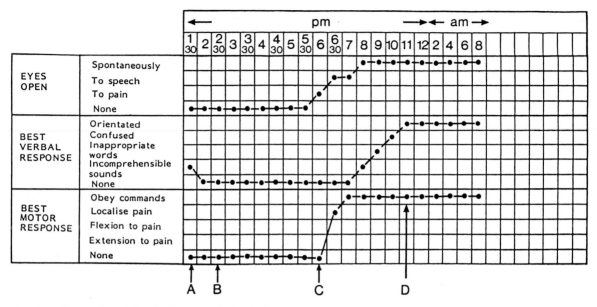

Fig. 5.7 Example of the influence of alcohol.

A 50 year old man was found lying in the street with abrasions of his forehead and smelling of alcohol. During the ambulance journey to hospital he was able to talk but on arrival his verbal response had deteriorated (A). He was breathing satisfactorily, had a normal pulse and blood pressure, no focal neurological signs and no evidence of extracranial injury.

A nasogastric tube, a bladder catheter and an intravenous cannula were inserted and he was placed in the recovery position. After half an hour he had no verbal response but his cardiorespiratory state remained stable.

Arterial blood gas analysis, blood glucose, serum electrolytes and X-rays of the cervical spine and skull were all within normal limits.

His blood alcohol level was 485 mg% (105 mmol/l).

A neurosurgeon was consulted one hour after admission (B) and advised that transfer was not appropriate at that stage. Three and a half hours later (C) his conscious level began to improve and five hours after that (D) he had regained full consciousness.

Thirty hours after arrival he had a grand mal seizure but subsequently made a good recovery.

orientation are usually restored within eight hours in most cases of alcohol intoxication (Fig. 5.8).

Deterioration

Apart from the closure of the eyes at night associated with sleep, any depression of the eye opening, verbal or motor response which are noted by a nurse warrants immediate notification of a doctor. Should this be confirmed by the doctor and no other cause be found (hypoglycaemia, anoxia, drug abuse) then the neurosurgeon should be contacted regarding treatment of a possible intracranial haematoma. The same concern should apply to a patient who

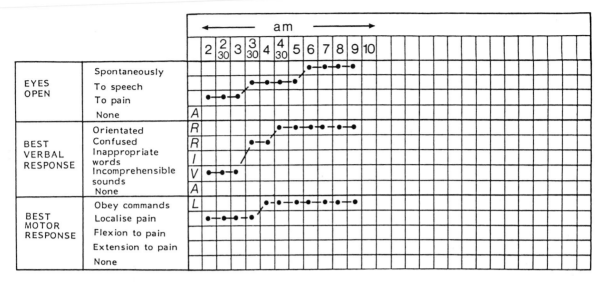

Fig. 5.8 Another example of the influence of alcohol.

A 25 year old woman fell while under the influence of alcohol, suffering a laceration of the forehead. She had no skull fracture and no focal neurological signs but she had vomited. When examined eight hours after arrival she was fully conscious and had no complaints but was a little tremulous. She was advised to remain until a relative arrived but she took her own discharge.

develops a focal neurological deficit or worsening of an existing deficit. If neurosurgery is thought to be necessary, the airway should be secured, ventilation restored, and an i.v. cannula inserted. A dose of 1g/kg of 20% Mannitol should be given over 10–15 min (i.e about 300–400 ml for an adult) or an 80 mg bolus of Frusemide only if agreed by the neurosurgeon. This will hopefully reduce the intracranial pressure and minimize secondary brain damage while transfer to a neurosurgical theatre is expedited (Section 4.2).

Sometimes 'deterioration' is due to a combination of delayed absorption of alcohol, fatigue and the head injury. Alcohol must never be the first thought of the staff when reviewing such a patient (Fig. 5.9) and the nursing staff should always consult the doctor in every case. Unless the conscious level can be quickly restored an urgent CT scan is indicated. Fig. 5.10 shows an example where alcohol was found to be the only cause of deterioration.

Epilepsy

If a fit follows a head injury in a non-epileptic patient, this is an indication for neurosurgical consultation. A single fit in a known epileptic does not warrant urgent neurosurgical referral provided there is good neurological recovery and skull fracture has been excluded.

Most people will recover from an epileptic fit within an hour or so but if the fit is secondary to acute brain damage, in

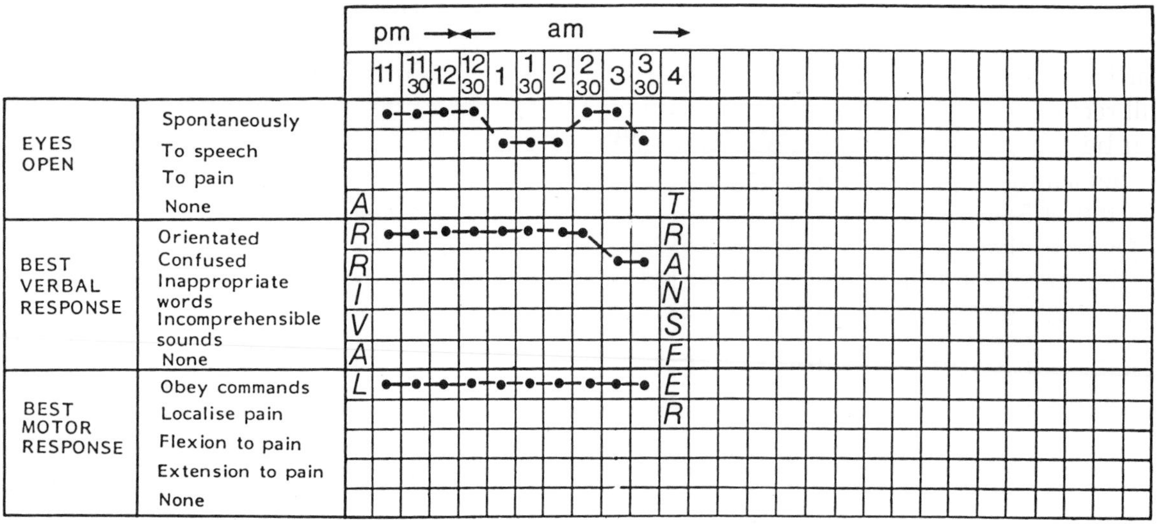

Fig. 5.9 Glasgow Coma Scale observation chart — times pm → ← am: 11, 11:30, 12, 12:30, 1, 1:30, 2, 2:30, 3, 3:30, 4. Left margin (vertical): ARRIVAL. Right margin (vertical): TRANSFERRED.

		EYES OPEN
EYES OPEN	Spontaneously	
	To speech	
	To pain	
	None	
BEST VERBAL RESPONSE	Orientated	
	Confused	
	Inappropriate words	
	Incomprehensible sounds	
	None	
BEST MOTOR RESPONSE	Obey commands	
	Localise pain	
	Flexion to pain	
	Extension to pain	
	None	

Fig. 5.9 Example of the association of alcohol and an extradural haematoma.

A 21 year old man was involved in a fight in a public house. He suffered a closed linear fracture of the right parietal region of the skull. Four hours after arrival in A and E he became disorientated in time and place. The resident doctor was immediately called and urgent transfer to the neurosurgery unit arranged. A right-sided extradural haematoma was evacuated. The patient made a full recovery.

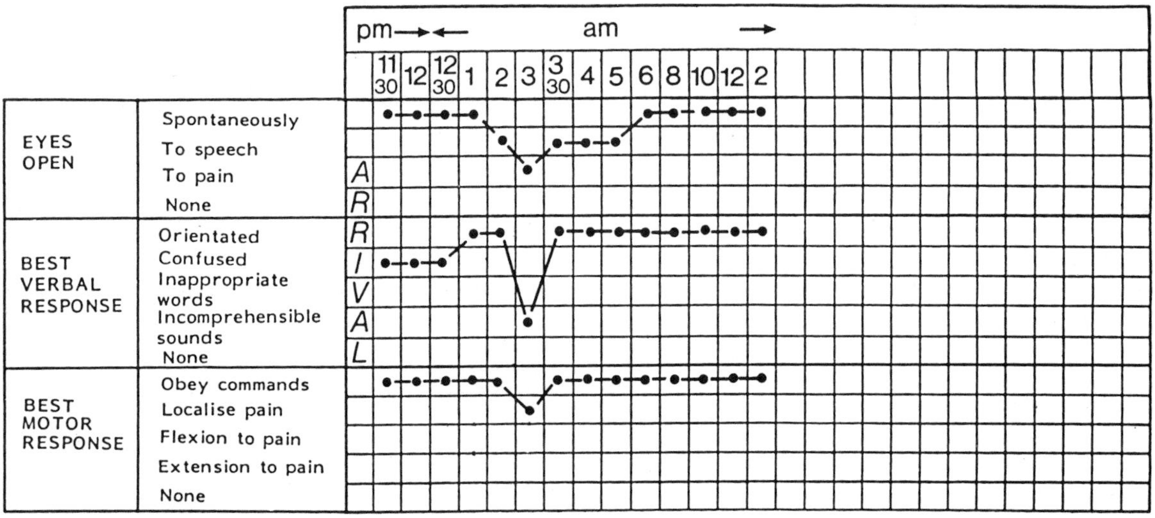

Fig. 5.10 Glasgow Coma Scale observation chart — times pm → ← am: 11:30, 12, 12:30, 1, 2, 3, 3:30, 4, 5, 6, 8, 10, 12, 2. Left margin (vertical): ARRIVAL.

		EYES OPEN
EYES OPEN	Spontaneously	
	To speech	
	To pain	
	None	
BEST VERBAL RESPONSE	Orientated	
	Confused	
	Inappropriate words	
	Incomprehensible sounds	
	None	
BEST MOTOR RESPONSE	Obey commands	
	Localise pain	
	Flexion to pain	
	Extension to pain	
	None	

Fig. 5.10 A further example of the influence of alcohol.

A 17 year old boy was assaulted on a Saturday night outside a public house. He was brought to the A and E department by police because he had a scalp laceration. On arrival he was found to be smelling strongly of alcohol, had slurred speech and was not sure what had happened.

There was no fracture detected either on wound exploration or on skull X-ray and he had no other abnormal neurological findings. On the observation ward, one and a half hours after arrival in A and E, he became orientated but two hours later the nurse found that his conscious level had deteriorated. This was an isolated observation and the resident doctor did not need to contact a neurosurgeon. The boy was fit to go home 15 hours after arrival.

particular raised intracranial pressure, then full recovery may not occur and the patient can be left with a focal neurological deficit or persisting depression in conscious level (Section 4.3).

During the fit, intravenous diazepam emulsion (Diazemuls) 10 mg can be given and if control is not obtained the dose should be repeated. If status epilepticus supervenes, maintenance of ventilation and oxygenation is most important and the services of an anaesthetist may be required.

If the patient is a known epileptic (or if in doubt) it is important to take a blood sample to check the anticonvulsant level(s) as sometimes the cause of the fit is the toxic effect of the anticonvulsant. Thereafter prophylactic anticonvulsant therapy can be given, e.g. intravenous phenytoin 250–750 mg slowly (50 mg/min) with ECG control.

Two or more 'moderate risk factors'

Rather than waiting for deterioration to become evident, the presence of an expanding intracranial haematoma may be anticipated by urgently referring patients with two or more of the following features:

- Skull fracture
- Depressed conscious level
- Focal neurological signs
- Constant severe headache
- Repeated vomiting after admission

Criteria for less urgent consultation with a neurosurgeon

1. Continuing depression of conscious level

When there is residual depression of conscious level, even if this is merely disorientation, after eight hours of observation, this means that the patient should be referred. This rule should apply even if there has been a heavy intake of alcohol prior to the head injury (hypoglycaemia should also be excluded). Persistent vomiting, severe constant headache unrelieved by simple analgesia, or residual focal signs after eight hours should all prompt discussion of the situation with a neurosurgeon.

2. Fractured base of skull

Neurosurgeons are particularly interested in patients where CSF leak persists beyond one week as neurosurgery may be required to close a dural defect. They have a vested interest in correct initial management and may wish to transfer such patients to ensure strict bed rest, antibiotic therapy and care of potential complications, e.g. facial palsy or meningitis. Signs of meningeal irritation such as photophobia, neck stiffness, Kernig's sign and pyrexia, may indicate infection or traumatic subarachnoid haemorrhage. In either case lumbar puncture should not be performed in the A and E department. The intracranial pressure may be raised. Let the neurosurgeons take responsibility for the consequences!

3. Depressed skull fracture

If there is any doubt about the nature of a fracture on wound exploration or stand-

—— (continued) ——

(continued)

and skull X-rays then tangential views are valuable to determine the presence and extent of the depression. Wounds should be thoroughly cleaned, severe bleeding stopped by suturing the skin, antibiotics commenced, oral fluids withheld and transfer arranged when mutually convenient. Closed depressed fractures are less common and unlikely to require operative intervention, but the radiographs should be shown to a neurosurgeon.

5.5 TRANSFER TO THE NEUROSURGERY DEPARTMENT

The number of referrals between A and E and neurosurgery is influenced by many factors, geographical, organizational and historical, as well as clinical. However it is our general experience that about 2% of patients arriving in the A and E department with a head injury will be referred for neurosurgical advice. In the UK this usually involves transfer by ambulance. The majority will be sent directly from the resuscitation area, or the observation ward.

It is essential that urgent referrals are adequately prepared. A final check should be made to exclude extracranial causes of cerebral deterioration (Section 4.1), the airway immaculately maintained and a good intravenous line established. About one fifth will be in coma and many will require endotracheal intubation and ventilation prior to transfer. A doctor and nurse should always accompany the patient when the latter's condition is unstable – and it usually will be as that is the commonest reason for referral. They must be able to maintain a good airway and carry appropriate equipment and drugs. These are listed in Table 5.3.

The form reproduced in Fig. 5.11 acts as a useful checklist for the referring hospital (which retains a copy) and provides valuable information for the receiving hospital to

Table 5.3 Contents of a patient transfer box

Intravenous fluids
Sodium chloride 0.9%
Haemaccel or Gelofusin
Sodium bicarbonate 8.4%
Mannitol 20%

Drugs
All to be given intravenously except Stesolid.
Diazepam emulsion
Stesolid (rectal diazepam)
Phenytoin
Frusemide
50% dextrose
Naloxone (adult and neonatal)
Atropine*
Adrenaline 1:10 000*
Lignocaine 1%*
Hydrocortisone sodium phosphate

Equipment
Suction apparatus
Oro- and naso-pharyngeal airways
Oxygen cylinder and tubing
Face masks (polymask, for 100% oxygen)
Ambu bag
Endotracheal tubes, laryngoscope etc.
Portable ventilator
Monitor/defibrillator
Intravenous cannulae and infusion sets
Needles and syringes
Swabs, bandages and tape and scissors

* May also be given via the endotracheal tube.

```
┌─────────────────────────────────────────────────────────────────────────┐
│                 HEAD INJURY TRANSFER CHECK LIST                            │
│                                                                            │
│  NAME:................................    M  ☐  F  ☐   D.O.B.  /  /        │
│  ADDRESS..............................    HOSPITAL NO.....................  │
│                                           RELIGION.......................  │
│  NEXT OF KIN:................................... NOT KNOWN           ☐      │
│  NOTIFIED:  NO  ☐   YES  ☐                TELEPHONE NO:................... │
│  VALUABLES:.......................         CLOTHING:.....................  │
│  REASON(S) FOR TRANSFER:                  DETERIORATING CONSCIOUS LEVEL ☐  │
│                                           SEIZURE(S)                   ☐   │
│                                           COMPOUND DEPRESSED SKULL FRACT ☐ │
│                                           FOR C.T. SCAN               ☐    │
│                                           OTHER.....................  ☐    │
│  MAJOR EXTRA CRANIAL INJURY (WARRANTING ADMISSION):  CERVICAL SPINE ☐ CHEST ☐ │
│  ABDOMEN ☐ PELVIS ☐ LIMB ☐ LUMBAR SPINE ☐ FACE ☐ OTHER____NONE    ☐      │
│  PAST ILLNESS & MEDICATION:.....................................          │
│  .................................................. NONE KNOWN     ☐      │
│  DRUGS GIVEN.....................................................         │
│  .......................................................... NONE    ☐     │
│  TETANUS PROPHYLAXIS:              ATT ☐   HATI ☐   NONE            ☐      │
│                                                                            │
│  AIRWAY:   GUEDEL ☐ ET. TUBE ☐ OTHER ☐.................... NONE    ☐      │
│  VENTILATION.: AMBU. BAG ☐ PORTABLE VENTILATER ☐   SPONTANEOUS      ☐      │
│  OXYGEN:     100% ☐    24% ☐   OTHER ☐............ AIR              ☐      │
│  I/V CANNULA IN SITU:           YES ☐               NO             ☐       │
│  BLOOD X MATCHED:   YES ☐ ...................UNITS  NO             ☐       │
│  N/G TUBE IN SITU:              YES ☐               NO             ☐       │
│  VOMITED:                       YES ☐               NO             ☐       │
│  CATHETER IN SITU:              YES ☐               NO             ☐       │
│  POSITION:   SUPINE ☐ LATERAL ☐     OTHER ☐.................               │
│  ARTERIAL BLOOD GASES   NO ☐   YES ☐ pO₂ .........mmHg  pCO₂ .......mmHg   │
│  BLOOD PRESSURE..............mmHg    PULSE RATE.............../min.         │
│  COMA SCALE ON TRANSFER    EYES_____ MOTOR_____ VERBAL_____            │
│  ESCORT:        ANAESTHETIST ☐  A/E DOCTOR ☐  NURSE               ☐        │
│  PHOTOCOPY OF NOTES: ☐   CHARTS ☐ X-RAYS ☐  DOCTORS LETTER        ☐        │
│  DATE  /  / .        Time of Transfer............................          │
│  FROM      WARD 45/46 ☐ A/E Resuscitation Area ☐ I.T.U. ☐ OTHER   ☐       │
│  Signature of Doctor in Charge...................................          │
│  Signature of Nurse in Charge....................................          │
│                                                    Fairfield/SW/22187      │
└─────────────────────────────────────────────────────────────────────────┘
```

Fig. 5.11 A head injury transfer checklist.

supplement the doctor's letter and verbal information.

5.6 HEAD INJURY ADVICE

When any head injured patient is allowed home, either from the A and E department or from the observation ward, he or she should be accompanied by a relative or other responsible adult who should be advised of the changes in the patient's condition which would warrant urgent review at the A and E department. Ideally a head injury warning card should be given to this adult as a reminder of these features (Fig. 4.10; Section 4.6). Some patients do not have access to a telephone or transport and may have no fixed abode, sleeping in conditions where deterioration would be

---

Box 5

CASE HISTORY

A seventy-five year old widow was found lying in the hall one morning by her home help. On arrival at the Accident and Emergency Department she was confused but had no other neurological signs or symptoms. There were abrasions of her nose and forehead. Her pulse rate was 60/minute and BP 120/70. She appeared clinically to be mildly dehydrated but examination of the chest and abdomen was unremarkable. X-rays of skull and cervical spine showed no fracture. X-rays of pelvis and hips showed degeneration changes only. The ECG was normal.

What is your immediate management?

- Referral to GP and Social Services for community support?
- Admission to short stay ward for observation?
- Further investigation in A and E?

This lady had fallen the previous evening and was now mildly hypothermic. Rectal temperature was 33°C. Blood sugar was normal. Other possibilities include chronic subdural haematoma (CT scan) and chest infection with hypoxia (blood gases).

She became fully orientated after gradual rewarming and was admitted to the short stay ward for observation. The health visitor was alerted and steps were taken to try to avoid a repetition of the incident after the patient had been discharged home.

Golden rule

Always check the temperature of a confused patient with a low reading thermometer.

unlikely to be noticed. It is reasonable to offer such patients overnight accommodation in a short stay ward, particularly if they present during the night. During working hours the hospital social worker may be able to arrange suitable accommodation in the community.

Patients may not be prepared to wait for a friend or relative to accompany them home, in which case this fact should be documented and witnessed and the patient should at least be given appropriate advice and the head injury warning card. In the unfortunate situation where deterioration occurs and the patient is not capable of seeking help, then the card may still be of value in speeding up the appropriate referral and therapy. How (it may be asked)

can this happen if our policy for admission is correct? Suffice to say that even if the policy is perfect it is impossible to ensure that it is completely understood and reliably enforced on all occasions.

Although the head injury warning advice is mainly intended to cover the 24 hours following discharge, it should be explained that symptoms such as prolonged or severe headache or confusion which occur in the following six weeks could possibly be related to the head injury and warrant review at the hospital. Subacute or chronic subdural haematomas may occur without a skull fracture in elderly patients and the initial findings may not be sufficient to warrant admission.

6 Follow-up and rehabilitation

Early recovery from the physical, psychological and social effects of minor head injury depends on appropriate care before, during and after attendance at the Accident and Emergency department. The A and E doctor is rightly concerned with detecting potentially life-threatening conditions including acute intracranial haematoma and compound skull fracture, but the potential morbidity associated with the apparently mild injury must also be recognized. This can include delayed healing of a scalp laceration due to a retained foreign body and infection, neuritis and cosmetic deformity. Persisting neurological and psychological symptoms and other medical problems may predispose the patient to further accidents.

Treatment therefore embraces the exclusion of major injury, attention to detail in the management of the small wound, and appropriate advice on rehabilitation and prevention.

6.1 RETURN PATIENTS

Most patients who are discharged from the A and E department after initial presentation or a short period of observation can resume normal activities after a few days spent quietly at home. However, about 3% return to the Accident and Emergency department within a few days or weeks of discharge. Their symptoms include headache, nausea, vomiting, dizziness, tiredness, irritability and forgetfulness. The underlying cause of each symptom may be different – either organic or psychological in origin – and is sometimes coincidental to the original injury.

The main concern of the casualty officer should be to exclude a serious complication of the head injury, e.g. an acute or chronic intracranial haematoma or infection. It is therefore essential to carry out a thorough neurological assessment. If the history or physical findings are at all suggestive of raised intracranial pressure or intracranial infection then admission for observation and further investigation is essential. This will usually be arranged in consultation with the appropriate in-patient specialty.

If repeated observations fail to detect any positive neurological signs, and particularly if the symptoms are intermittent and improving with rest, then further assessment in the out-patient department may be appropriate. The routine referral of such patients to a 'head injury follow-up clinic' has certain advantages. It allows the effectiveness of initial management to be monitored and gives some insight into the natural progression of so-called 'minor' head injury. The clinic also provides an opportunity for teaching doctors and nurses about the often significant consequences of such injuries. Most importantly, the clinic encourages an early multidisciplinary approach to patient management which many consider to be essential for successful treatment.

Just as with the rehabilitation of severely head injured patients, it may be necessary to work closely with the clinical psychologist, ENT surgeon, ophthalmologist, physiotherapist and social worker. Help and advice may be required at short notice. Ideally, there should be a flexible arrangement, allowing the patient to be seen by several specialists on the same day.

6.2 PRESENTING SYMPTOMS

Headache

Patients with unexplained symptoms are quite naturally concerned, and headache is a particularly emotive symptom. On most occasions when patients return to the Accident and Emergency department complaining of headache this will be due at least in part to the head injury. It is worth re-emphasizing the importance of first excluding intracranial haematoma (Section 5.4) and infection (Section 5.4) even at this late stage.

Extracerebral causes of headache must then be considered. Sometimes the headache is localized to the site of the scalp wound. If this occurs within a few days of injury, infection of the wound is a possibility (Section 6.6). Pain or paraesthesia radiating from the site of a healing or healed wound may be described as 'sharp', 'shooting', 'tingling', a 'tight or numb feeling' or 'like running water'. These symptoms are usually due to damaged cutaneous nerves and are associated with altered or absent sensation in the skin supplied (Figs 4.4 and 4.5). Percussion of the scar or tender area of the scalp often reproduces paraesthesia and headache. This sensitivity should lessen with time and can be helped by encouraging normal palpation of the scalp and regular massage of the tender area. If the pain is severe and persistent then the opinion of a plastic surgeon should be sought although excision of a 'neuroma' is rarely necessary.

Headaches attributed to 'tension' or 'muscle contraction' are perhaps the commonest type. They are usually bilateral, affecting the fronto-temporal or occipital region, dull in nature, and often described as a feeling of pressure or like a 'band around the head'. They have usually been experienced on occasions prior to the head injury, become worse as the day progresses and are not relieved significantly by analgesics. A psychologist may be able to help these patients by assessing their social and psychological stresses and by giving relaxation therapy.

Head injury may lead to an increase in frequency and severity of attacks in migraine sufferers. Typically there is a unilateral headache associated with nausea and lasting for several hours or days. The patient should be reminded to avoid alcohol, cheese, chocolate and other dietary trigger factors. Simple analgesics, e.g. paracetamol, should be prescribed together with an anti-emetic. Long term prophylactic treatment, e.g. Propranolol (Inderal) should be continued until reviewed by the general practitioner.

Sometimes headaches develop which are completely coincidental to the injury. Some of these are short-lived and others respond to simple treatment, of, for example an upper respiratory tract infection, dental abscess and sinusitis. Persisting headaches warrant further investigation to exclude important conditions such as cerebral tumours, temporal arteritis and glaucoma.

Headaches situated in the occipital region radiating to the fronto-temporal region or behind the eye may be due to neck strain with cervical nerve root irritation. If there are associated neck symptoms then treatment should be directed accordingly.

Neck pain

Neck symptoms usually develop following a flexion/extension injury without any obvious fracture or dislocation evident on X-ray. Typically the stiffness and pain become significant several hours or days after the injury and may be associated with intermittent paraesthesiae radiating to one or both hands. Radiology of the cervical spine (Section 3.3) is essential not only to exclude bony injury but also to demonstrate features which may contribute to symptoms, e.g. cervical spondylosis or cervical rib. Patients with neurological signs should be referred for orthopaedic or neurosurgical advice. Treatment for the remainder, who form the majority of patients, includes a well-fitting supporting collar which is worn initially both at night and during the day. If symptoms do not begin to respond within a few days of resting in a collar, and providing there are no neurological signs, then gentle massage, heat and exercise under the direction of a physiotherapist should help speed recovery.

Dizziness and vertigo

The patient with vestibular mechanism disturbance usually complains of vertigo induced by positional change of the head, e.g. on turning or looking up quickly. Enquiry should be made to exclude other causes of the dizziness, e.g. antihypertensive therapy, alcohol abuse, cervical spine problems and previous ear trouble. The blood pressure should be checked. The neck should be examined for movement, tenderness and the presence of a carotid bruit.

The finding of positionally induced nystagmus using Cawthorne's Test (Fig. 2.9; Section 2.8) distinguishes true vertigo from other types of dizziness (Table 1.1; Section 1.4). In all but the mildest cases, it is wise to refer patients with vertigo to an ENT surgeon at an early stage to exclude a treatable cause, e.g. leakage of labyrinthine fluid.

In patients without specific organic disease it is difficult to predict the prognosis. This can only be determined over a period of months by repeated examination. Betahistine tablets (8 mg taken 8 hourly) may alleviate symptoms, but it has to be admitted that any improvement is usually spontaneous. The patient will learn to adapt his or her behaviour to reduce the residual symptom. Positional testing has a 'fatiguing effect', vertigo and nystagmus tending to be diminished on repeated testing. This can be used therapeutically if the patient carries out positional exercises several times each day.

Vomiting

Children are sometimes brought back to the Accident and Emergency department because they have started vomiting for the first time a few days after a head injury. Usually this is due to a coincidental infection but, especially in the young child, admission is the safest way of being sure. Observation in an isolation ward is prudent if diarrhoea or contagious disease is suspected. The temperature should be checked, the respiratory tract examined and urinalysis and urine culture carried out. A close watch should be kept for a rash.

Providing neurological observations are satisfactory, or if there is convincing evidence of nothing more than a simple viral infection, the child is often best nursed at home. Persistent nausea or vomiting will demand specialist referral. However, it is very unlikely that this will be the only symptom associated with deteriorating neurological status. Similarly, vomiting in a fully conscious adult without neurological signs is likely to be due to a coincidental condition, e.g. gastritis or peptic ulcer.

Otorrhoea

The leakage of clear fluid from the ear should be assumed to be cerebro-spinal fluid coming from a basal skull fracture until proved otherwise. Management of the latter is discussed in Section 5.4. Other causes include otitis externa precipitated by local trauma or the serum from blood which has run into the canal from a scalp wound. If there is doubt about the nature of the discharge then an immediate ENT opinion must be obtained and sufficient fluid collected for bacteriological and biochemical analysis (Section 3.2). An auroscope should be used with caution as it may introduce infection. A detailed examination should

not be undertaken in the A and E department if a basal skull fracture cannot be excluded.

Rhinorrhoea

A patient may return complaining that he has had clear fluid leaking from the nose. If this is associated with a recent frontal fracture then it is essential to commence antibiotics, carry out a brow-up lateral skull X-ray (to exclude an aerocoele: Section 4.2), and discuss further management with a neurosurgeon.

If there is no evidence of a recent fracture, the patient is well and fluid cannot be obtained by a provocation test (head down with pressure on the jugular veins) then out-patient management may be appropriate. The patient should be given universal containers and asked to return with a specimen as soon as fluid is produced. Sometimes the cause is serum escaping from an organized clot associated with a nasal fracture, an incidental allergic rhinitis or simply a 'cold'.

Anosmia

Loss of the sense of smell impairs taste discrimination. Patients who claim that 'their food now tastes different' are usually suffering from anosmia.

Total anosmia after head injury is caused by injury to the first nerve projections across the cribriform plate. These can be considered to be part of the central nervous system rather than peripheral nerves, and repair does not occur. Repeated testing over several weeks may be of value to exclude those with temporary impairment due to rhinitis. Complete anosmia persisting for a year is likely to be permanent.

It is not generally appreciated that anosmia is a relatively common sequel to head injury. Many patients find it a significant disability. They should be warned about their inability to detect hazards such as escaping gas and fumes.

Visual problems

Some patients attend opticians to have their eyes 'tested' after a head injury because of frontal headaches or because they think their eyesight has deteriorated. If they find that their visual acuity is impaired then they may assume that this is due to the head injury. This is rarely the case and usually represents the exposure of a pre-existing impairment.

In contrast, temporary re-activation of a strabismus commonly occurs following a deceleration type of injury. Whether this is due to physical damage or emotional stress is not known. Delayed onset of ptosis and isolated paresis of extra-ocular muscles has also been described unassociated with demonstrable intracranial pathology. Once the latter has been excluded the patient can be reassured that motor function will return spontaneously. However, full recovery may take up to two years.

Facial palsy

When a lower motor neurone facial weakness (Section 2.10) has been observed to develop some days after a fracture of the petrous temporal bone has been sustained,

recovery is likely within three months. If however the palsy was noted immediately after the injury, it is possible that the facial nerve has been severed in its bony canal. In this case an ENT opinion should be sought regarding repair. In all patients with persisting facial palsy, tarsorrhaphy to protect the eye should be considered.

6.3 PSYCHOLOGICAL SYMPTOMS

Often the cause of headache and dizziness is not immediately apparent to the busy casualty officer. The patient is quite reasonably reluctant to discuss psychological complaints in the midst of a busy A and E department but these may be the main reason for his attendance (Table 6.1). In this case a brief enquiry about 'sleep disturbance, tiredness and irritability' should help to identify the need for a fuller interview in more appropriate conditions.

Symptoms such as poor concentration and forgetfulness may be due to genuine, albeit temporary, organic brain damage with difficulty in processing information [10]. This disability, as well as the physical effects of the head injury, may lead to a change in self-image, to a lack of self-confidence and consequently to an exacerbation of psychological symptoms. In most cases these symptoms resolve within a few weeks. However, if they do not, social and psychological factors become increasingly important including the pre-morbid personality and support (or lack of it) received from family, friends and health care professionals.

Full psychological assessment is time-

Table 6.1 Frequency of neurological and psychological symptoms 1–3 weeks after mild head injury. (Compiled from a survey of 32 patients with post-traumatic amnesia less than 12 hours, and selected to exclude those with previous psychological disturbance.)

Psychological	%	Neurological
	80	Headache
	70	
Tiredness		
	60	
Irritability; loss of drive		
Sleep disturbance	50	
		Dizziness
	40	
Tension		
Restlessness		
Poor concentration	30	
Depression; Inattention		
Shakiness; Low alcohol tolerance	20	Impaired hearing
Incompetence; Sweating		
Forgetfulness; Panic attacks		Tinnitus
	10	Neck pain; Visual disturbance; Anosmia
Loss of libido		
Loss of emotion		Slurred speech; Unsteadiness

consuming and is best left to a clinical psychologist. However, use of a checklist of common psychological symptoms together with simple tests of cognitive function (the serial 7 subtraction test and the ability to remember an address) should enable the non-specialist to recognize those patients requiring further assessment. The psychologist will assess the attitudes, needs, strengths and weaknesses of a patient's current level of functioning. Cognitive, behavioural and emotive changes will be monitored and an attempt will be made to differentiate psychiatric symptoms from those which could be due to 'brain damage'.

Exacerbating factors

- Lack of early informed advice on the meaning of symptoms. Patients may be convinced that the presence of a

(continued)

(continued)

headache indicates serious intracranial pathology. Sometimes they have friends or relatives who have undergone neurosurgery or suffered a serious head injury. It may be a great relief for them to learn that a headache, for example, is not of such a serious nature.

- The stress of returning to work and resuming normal activities may reveal that the patient has not fully recovered from the head injury. This in itself can cause further anxiety and may exacerbate the symptoms.
- A previous tendency to migraine or headaches may be associated with particularly severe or prolonged headaches following a minor head injury.
- Alcohol or drug abuse. Patients may discover that they have a lowered tolerance when they resume their habit.
- Recall of the accident or assault which caused the head injury may in itself be a source of anxiety or depression.
- The stress of legal proceedings may sharpen the patient's awareness of his symptoms. This may be manifest by the recurrence of symptoms a year or more after the injury when the patient and his lawyer are preparing for the case to go to court. There is no evidence, however, that successful litigation is associated with resolution of symptoms. It is unwise and unkind to assume that the patient's symptoms are magnified by avarice.

6.4 TREATMENT

Much of the anxiety associated with head injury and the resultant exacerbation of symptoms can be avoided by appropriate treatment. This should include counselling in the A and E department, during the patient's hospital stay and by follow-up in a clinic where time is available for a thorough neuropsychological assessment. Patients should be advised that they may not be able to cope immediately with demanding activities and that premature return to work or sport can precipitate new symptoms. There is evidence that advice including bed rest for one week after the injury will markedly reduce the incidence of psychological sequelae, particularly in those under 60 years of age [11].

So-called 'leisure activities' can be as harmful as work to those with impaired ability to process information. Watching television, particularly while attempting to carry out other activities, is stressful. Conversation in a crowded room (such as a bar!) is difficult at the best of times. Alcohol tolerance may be reduced and as its effects can mimic or add to those of the head injury it is best avoided. As a general rule activities demanding rapid responses and a high level of co-ordination should be avoided for at least two weeks after even a brief period of post-traumatic amnesia. A gradual return to full activities should be encouraged, providing there are no residual problems. Some sporting bodies have their own recommendations. For example, the International Rugby Football Board advocates a minimum of three weeks off after 'concussion' has been diagnosed and most boxing authorities recommend at least four weeks' rest from sparring after a contest has been stopped due to head injury. Perhaps similar constraints should be suggested for driving and cycling.

Sexual problems, usually loss of libido, are the source of much anxiety but are rarely presenting complaints. They are usually psychological in origin and the patient can be reassured that they will improve in time as the other symptoms resolve.

The psychologist employs behaviour techniques for anxiety, phobias, cognitive distortions and lowered self-image. The use of relaxation therapy can avoid excessive prescription of tranquillizing medication. Occasionally however when a patient has suicidal thoughts, hallucinations or other psychotic symptoms, a psychiatrist's opinion is more appropriate.

6.5 RELATIVES

The support of understanding relatives, friends and employers can make a great contribution to the rehabilitation of a head injured patient. It is helpful for a relative to attend the follow-up clinic no matter what the age of the patient.

The frank opinion of a close relative will often reveal psychological and relevant social problems that may not be volunteered by a patient. Sometimes the spouse notices changes in the patient's personality of which he or she is not aware. Agreement on symptoms by patient and relative when interviewed separately is also helpful in building up an accurate picture of psychological problems.

Relatives can help remind patients with poor short-term memory or weak will to heed the doctor's advice in such matters as rest, taking regular medication and abstaining from alcohol. The stress of caring for such patients has been recognized by the establishment of the 'Headway' organization. Groups meet regularly throughout Great Britain offering advice and support to relatives of head injured patients. Further information can be obtained from Headway (National Head Injuries Association), 200 Mansfield Road, Nottingham NG1 3HX (telephone 0602 622382).

6.6 WOUND INFECTION

Scalp wounds heal remarkably well because of their good blood supply. Infection usually occurs in a neglected wound. Either there has been delay in seeking medical help or there has been inadequate wound toilet. Minor or local infection can usually be managed by thorough wound debridement and excision of all dirt and necrotic tissue. Sutures are removed where necessary and the wound allowed to granulate up and close by secondary intention. Wound management is described in detail in Section 4.4.

With more significant infection, the patient complains of a throbbing pain within a few days of injury. There may be peri-orbital swelling, even when the wound is well behind the frontal hair-line. If cellulitis is widespread the patient is usually febrile and will require admission (Fig. 6.1). All sutures should be removed to release pus which is usually staphylococcal in origin. Sometimes there is only a little watery pus, but much oedema and cellulitis, in which case a streptococcal infection should be suspected. Swabs should be taken and sent for immediate gram staining and culture. In a toxic patient (who is not allergic to penicillin) intravenous Penicillin G (1.2g., four-hourly) and intravenous Flucloxacillin (1 g, six-hourly) should be commenced, pending advice from a bacteriologist. Once the patient is fit for discharge, further

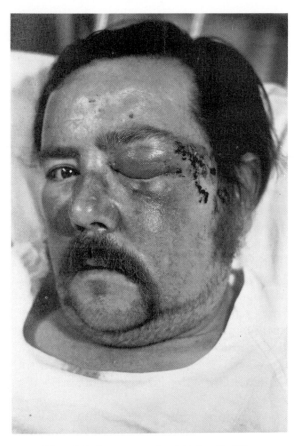

Fig. 6.1 Severe peri-orbital cellulitis.

management should include regular cleansing of the wound and shaving the surrounding skin.

Bone may be exposed after loss of necrotic skin. This is a major complication and the patient should be referred for a plastic surgeon's opinion. Early healing can be achieved by removal of the exposed outer table and application of a split skin graft. In the elderly and others with a thin skull it may be safer to apply regular dressings in which case it will take several months for

dead bone to sequestrate before the wound heals.

6.7 WORRYING BUMPS

The patient may be concerned about lumps and bumps. Some may have escaped the casualty officer's attention and some may have appeared subsequent to the Accident and Emergency attendance.

A scalp haematoma may be too tender initially to allow palpation. After a few days, as the oedema settles, the haematoma becomes softer with a well-defined edge. Palpation of this edge often gives the impression of a depressed fracture and, if there is doubt, tangential X-rays may be necessary to reassure doctor and patient (Fig. 2.2).

Large haematomas in young children are particularly worrying and may take several weeks to resolve. It is worthwhile making sequential measurements of the haematoma to reassure the parents that it is decreasing in size. Providing there is no cellulitis and the child is otherwise well then reassurance is all that is required.

Rarely, a pulsatile swelling of the scalp occurs in infants and toddlers some months after a fracture of the vault has been sustained. This is a due to a leakage of cerebrospinal fluid out through torn dura causing gradual separation of the bone edges (a 'growing fracture') and requires neurosurgical care.

Haematomas of the supra-orbital region can produce a temporary cosmetic problem. The lump may persist for several weeks but providing it is not infected, it is best left to resolve. A surgical incision would be more likely to lead to a permanent cosmetic

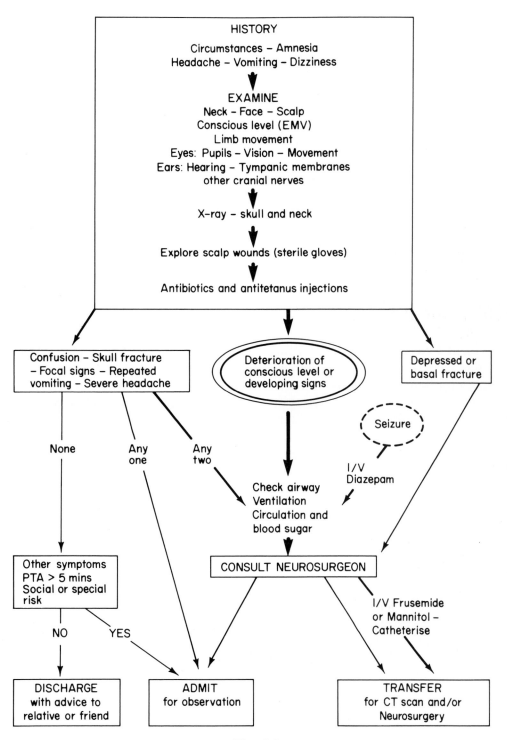

Fig. 6.2

problem and aspiration either fails or is followed by re-accumulation with the added risk of introducing infection.

Other bumps noticed by patients after head injuries range from occipital lymph nodes which can become enlarged following scalp injury to normal bony protuberances which have not previously been recognized.

Occasionally, some weeks after injury, foreign bodies such as glass fragments work their way to the surface. These may be difficult to differentiate from scar tissue until the tip of the foreign body causes irritation or bleeding and the site for retrieval become obvious.

6.8 THE 'AT-RISK PATIENT'

A fall or collapse resulting in a head injury may be related to a pre-existing illness, drug therapy for that illness or to a hitherto undiagnosed medical problem. These possibilities are particularly relevant to elderly patients. Appropriate investigation and treatment will reduce the risk of further incidents occurring.

Chronic alcohol and drug abusers often have social and psychological problems. Such patients are prone to accidents and assault and these usually involve the head. Admission to hospital can be the turning point in rehabilitation. The opportunity should not be missed to offer help to such patients in the form of counselling by a psychologist or social worker or referral to an alcohol or drug treatment centre. Occasionally a chronic alcoholic becomes a reformed character following head injury and proves the cynics wrong.

It may be possible to prevent some head injuries by health education. Nevertheless the mild head injury will continue to provide a huge workload which must be dealt with by commonsense measures. The action taken by first aiders and correct management in the Accident and Emergency department have longlasting effects and should pave the way for the gradual resumption of normal physical and mental activities. Table 6.2 summarizes the management advocated in earlier chapters and emphasizes the importance of an integrated response to this common problem.

Further reading

Jennett, B. and Teasdale, G. (1981) *Management of Head Injuries*, Davis, Philadelphia.

Potter, J. M. and Briggs, M. (1984) *The Practical Management of Head Injuries*, Lloyd Luke, London.

North, B. (1984) *Jamieson's First Notebook of Head Injury*, Butterworths, Sevenoaks, Kent.

Levin, H. (ed.) (1988) *Mild Head Injury*, Oxford University Press, Oxford.

References

1. Swann, I.J., MacMillan, R., and Strang, I. (1981) Head injuries at an inner city Accident and Emergency Department. *Injury*, **12**, 274–8.
2. Boulis Z.F., Dick R. and Barnes, N.R. (1978) Head injuries in children – aetiology, symptoms, physical findings and X-ray wastage. *Brit. J. Radiol.*, **51**, 851–4.
3. Fullarton, G.M., MacEwen, C.J., MacMillan, R. and Swann, I.J. (1987) An evaluation of open scalp wounds. *Arch. Emerg. Med.*, **4**, 11–16.
4. Teasdale, G. and Jennett, B. (1974) Assessment of coma and impaired consciousness. *Lancet* **ii**, 81–4
5. Mendelow, A.D., Karmi, M.Z., Paul, K.S., *et al.* (1979) Extradural haematoma: effect of delayed treatment. *Brit. Med. J.*, **1**, 1240–2.
6. *The Reduced Snellen's Chart.* Available from: Clement Clarke International Ltd., 16 Wigmore Street, London W1H ODH.
7. *Kay Picture Test (For Visual Acuity in Children).* Available from: P.O. Box 38, Bolton BL3 3TT.
8. Rose, J., Valtonen, S. and Jennett, B. (1977) Avoidable factors contributing to death after head injury. *Brit. Med. J.*, **2**, 615.
9. Group of Neurosurgeons (1984) Guidelines for the management of recent head injury in adults. *Brit. Med. J.* **288**, 983–5.
10. Gronwall, D. (1987) Advances in the assessment of attention and information processing after head injury, in *Neurobehavioural Recovery from Head Injury* (eds H.S. Levin, J. Grafman, H.M. Eisenberg), Oxford Unversity Press, Oxford.
11. Minderhoud, J.M., Boelens, M.E.M., Huizenea, J. and Saan, R.J. (1980) Treatment of minor head injuries. *Clin. Neurol. Neurosurg.*, **82**, 2.

Index